Type 2 Diabetes Cookbook for Women

Delicious Recipes and Lifestyle Strategies to Manage Blood Sugar and Enjoy Healthy Living

By

KELLY C. BROWN

Dear Readers,

Welcome to "Type 2 Diabetes Cookbook for Women".

I'm Kelly C. Brown, a dietitian deeply concerned for individuals health and well-being, with a focus on controlling type 2 diabetes via mindful eating. In this cookbook, I've compiled a variety of delectable dishes designed exclusively to aid women on their road to improved health and optimal blood sugar management.

As someone who is genuinely devoted to encouraging healthy living, I'm excited to provide you with a variety of tasty recipes tailored to your dietary requirements and tastes. Each recipe is carefully curated to not only please your taste sensations but also improve your overall health.

I've poured my heart and experience into this cookbook, and I truly believe it has the power to help you take charge of your health journey. As you read these pages, I urge you to seize the chance for good change and learn new methods to nurture your body and soul.

Your feedback is vital to me, as it will not only help me grow as an Author but also a guide for other readers looking to better their health. I kindly invite you to share your thoughts and experiences by leaving a review on Amazon, as your insights might inspire and help others to make informed choices about their well-being.

Thank you for choosing "Type 2 Diabetes Cookbook for Women".

Together, Let's go on a road to a better, more vibrant existence.

Warm regards.

Kelly C. Brown

Table of Contents

Introduction

Sarah felt sad with her Type 2 diabetes diagnosis. She was a little lost and didn't know where to start. One day while browsing an online bookstore she found a cookbook particularly developed for women with Type 2 diabetes.

Sarah was intrigued and grabbed up a copy. It was more than simply recipes, it was a guide to good eating. The book described how various foods affect blood sugar and provide clear instructions for meal preparation.

Week one was an eye-opener. Sarah switched from sweet breakfasts to fiber-rich porridge with berries. Lunch became a colorful salad with healthy protein, rather than a hefty sandwich. Dinners were a revelation of delicious stir-fries with veggies and lean proteins that didn't raise her blood sugar.

The cookbook became Sarah's regular companion. She uncovered hidden gems, such as diabetic-friendly muffins that filled her sweet appetite and veggie-packed lunches that helped her manage cravings. What is the best part? The meals were tasty.

Sarah sensed a shift over time. She had greater energy throughout the day, and lunchtime slumps were a distant memory. Regular blood sugar tests verified the good effect, with her readings progressively improving.

This was more than simply a diet, it was a lifestyle change. Sarah was equipped with the right knowledge she needed to know for her condition to make informed decisions. The cookbook served as a guide, but she had complete authority.

There were obstacles, of course. Birthday cake at work was tempting, but Sarah packed healthier options in her bag. Social events needed some forethought, but with the book's help, she was able to confidently navigate buffets and restaurant menus.

Sarah was not only managing her diabetes but flourishing as a result of her great meals and newly acquired knowledge. The cookbook was not a hindrance, but rather a doorway to a better, happier her.

Are you tired of bland, restrictive diets, and want to take charge of your health? This cookbook offers a tastier path to managing your blood sugar. Discover simple, flavorful recipes that help you feel great, all while keeping your health on track. This book empowers you with knowledge and delicious options, making healthy eating a joy, not a chore.

Chapter 1: Understanding Type 2 Diabetes

Welcome to a healthier you! This chapter is designed to empower you with knowledge about Type 2 Diabetes and confidence to manage the condition effectively.

What is Type 2 Diabetes?

Type 2 diabetes is a chronic illness in which your body struggles to control its blood sugar (glucose) levels. Imagine sugar as your body's fuel and insulin as the key that allows sugar to enter your cells. Type 2 diabetes occurs when your body does not create enough insulin or your cells develop resistance to its effects. If left untreated, sugar accumulation in the bloodstream may cause a variety of health concerns.

Factors Contributing to Type 2 Diabetes

Type 2 diabetes may affect everyone, but some things raise your risk. Understanding these elements allows you to take control of your health.

1. Weight: Being overweight, particularly around the abdomen, is a significant risk factor. Fat cells may develop resistance to insulin's actions.
2. Family History: Having a parent or sibling with type 2 diabetes raises your risk.
3. Ethnicity: Type 2 diabetes is more prevalent among African Americans, Hispanic/Latino Americans, Asian Americans, and Pacific Islanders.

4. Age: The chance of developing type 2 diabetes rises with age, although it may occur at any age.

5. Physical Inactivity: Regular exercise increases insulin sensitivity. A sedentary lifestyle raises your risk.

6. Diet: A diet heavy in processed foods, sugary drinks, and unhealthy fats may lead to insulin resistance.

7. Prediabetes: This is a condition in which blood sugar levels are above normal but not high enough to be diagnosed with type 2 diabetes. If left uncontrolled, it may lead to type 2 diabetes.

8. Gestational Diabetes: Having diabetes while pregnant increases your chances of acquiring type 2 diabetes later in life.

9. Polycystic Ovarian Syndrome (PCOS): This hormonal imbalance may impair insulin sensitivity.

The Impact of Type 2 Diabetes on the Body

When blood sugar levels rise steadily in type 2 diabetes, a domino effect occurs, affecting different organs and systems throughout the body. **Here's a close look:**

1. Blood Vessels: High blood sugar may cause blood vessels to stiffen and constrict. **This might lead to:**
    - Heart Disease: Reduced blood flow raises the risk of a heart attack or stroke.
    - Peripheral Artery Disease (PAD): Poor circulation in legs and feet may cause discomfort, and numbness, and raise the risk of infection.

- Kidneys: Overworked kidneys attempting to filter extra sugar can damage and develop kidney disease.

2. Eyes: Diabetic retinopathy is a condition in which high blood sugar destroys blood vessels in the retina, possibly resulting in visual loss.

3. Nerves: High blood sugar levels may damage nerves throughout the body, resulting in neuropathy. This might cause pain, tingling, numbness, and digestive difficulties.

4. Skin: Increased susceptibility to infections, sluggish wound healing, and skin issues may develop.

Signs and symptoms

Type 2 diabetes may creep up on you, causing symptoms to appear years later. However, your body often sends out early warning signals. **Here's what to look for:**

1. Increased Urination: One of the first indicators is frequent urination, particularly at night. Your body attempts to remove excess sugar via urine.

2. Excessive Thirst: As you lose fluids via frequent urine, your body gets dehydrated, resulting in acute thirst.

3. Extreme Hunger: Even if you are eating more, your cells are not receiving enough sugar for energy, resulting in persistent hunger sensations.

4. Unexplained Weight Loss: Despite eating more, your body struggles to utilize sugar for energy, resulting in unintentional weight loss.

5. Fatigue: Chronically high blood sugar levels may deplete your energy, leaving you exhausted and sluggish.

6. High blood sugar levels can cause blurry vision, slow wound healing, frequent yeast infections, itching, and dehydration.

7. Acanthosis nigricans cause velvety, darkened patches of skin on the back of the neck, armpits, and groin.

8. High blood sugar can cause nerve damage, resulting in numbness, tingling, or pain in the hands and feet.

How To Prevent and Manage Type 2 Diabetes

The good news is that type 2 diabetes may be mainly avoided and managed via healthy lifestyle choices. **Here are some ways to empower you:**

Diet:

1. Eat whole, unprocessed foods: Select fruits, vegetables, whole grains, lean proteins, and healthy fats. These give critical nutrients and help you feel fuller for longer, reducing blood sugar surges.

2. Limit sugary beverages and processed meals since they include refined carbs and added sugars, leading to a quick blood sugar increase.

3. Practice portion control by using smaller plates and bowls to prevent overeating.

4. Read food labels: Choose low-sugar alternatives.

5. Plan your meals and snacks: Avoid making bad choices when hungry.

Exercise:

1. Aim for at least 30 minutes of moderate-intensity activity on most days of the week: Brisk walking, swimming, cycling, and dancing are all great possibilities.

2. Find hobbies you like. Consistency is essential, so choose activities you will stay with.

3. Include strength training: Increasing muscle mass improves insulin sensitivity.

Weight Management:

1. Losing even a small amount of weight (5-7% of one's body weight) may considerably improve blood sugar management.

2. Prioritize healthy weight reduction via nutrition and exercise, avoiding fad diets.

Healthy Habits:

1. Get enough sleep: Aim for 7-8 hours of good sleep every night. Inadequate sleep may affect hormones that control blood sugar.

2. Managing stress: Chronic stress might cause elevated blood sugar levels. Practice relaxation methods such as yoga, meditation, and deep breathing.

3. Do not miss doctor's appointments: Regular visits let your doctor monitor your blood sugar levels and alter your treatment plan as required.

4. Stay informed: Learn about type 2 diabetes and its treatment. This enables you to make educated decisions regarding your health.

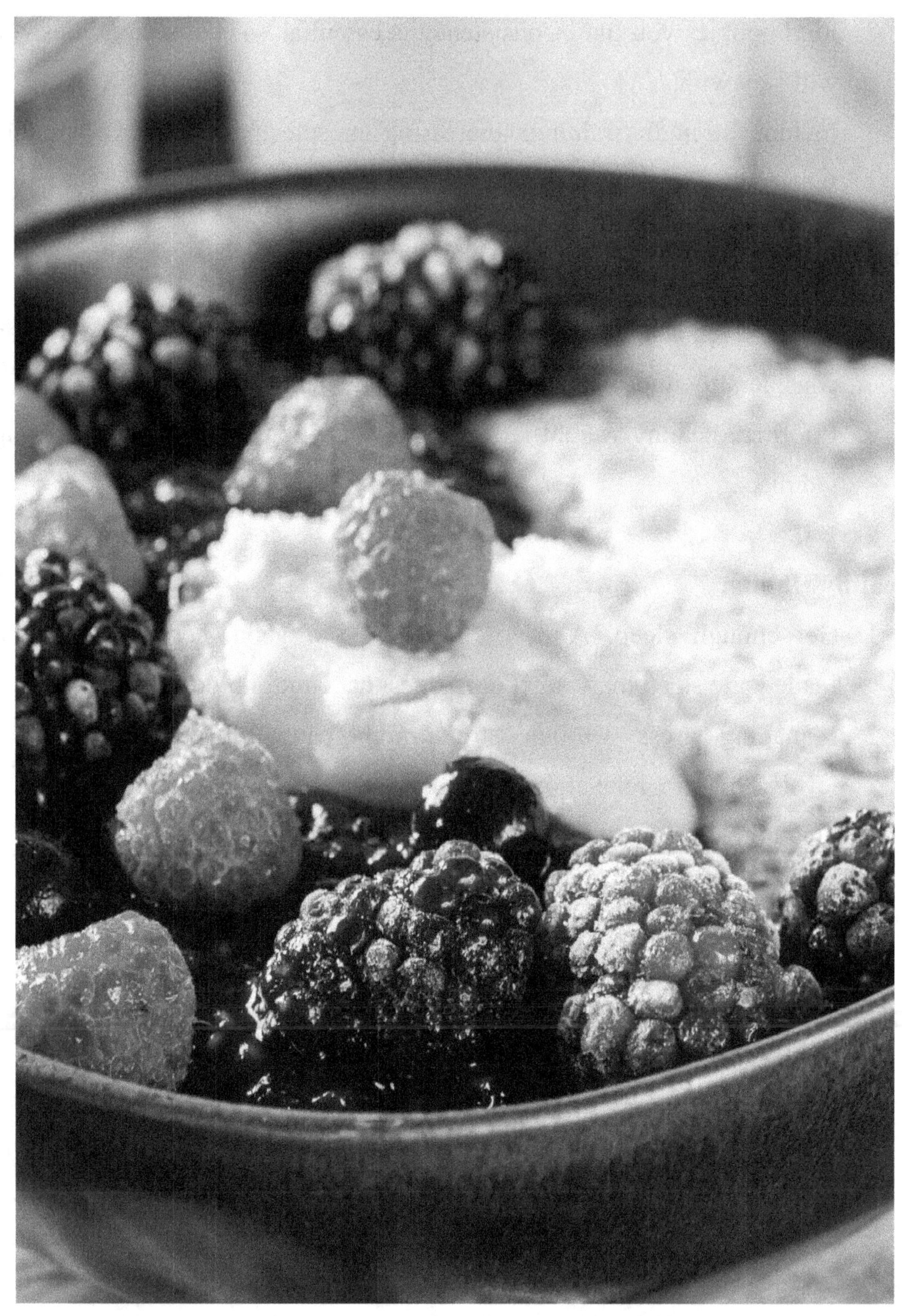

Chapter 2: Importance of Diet in Managing Type 2 Diabetes

While there is no cure for type 2 diabetes, a nutritious diet is the most effective way to manage blood sugar and improve your overall health. **Here's why:**

1. Blood Sugar Control: The carbs we consume convert into sugar. Choosing the correct meals and portion sizes may help manage blood sugar levels, reducing spikes and crashes.
2. Weight Management: Losing even a minor amount of weight may help with blood sugar management. Healthy eating encourages weight reduction and helps you maintain a healthy weight.
3. Reduced Risk of issues: Chronic high blood sugar levels may cause a variety of issues. A nutritious diet lowers the risk by improving blood sugar management.
4. Increased Energy Levels: Stable blood sugar levels deliver consistent energy throughout the day, allowing you to feel your best.
5. Overall health: A healthy diet rich in fruits, vegetables, whole grains, and lean protein contains important nutrients that promote general health and well-being.

This Cookbook Empowers You:

These pages provide excellent low-sugar recipes that help good blood sugar control. We'll show you how to make healthy, tasty meal choices.

Food is more than simply nourishment, it's an effective tool for controlling type 2 diabetes. Accept healthy eating as a means to take charge of your health and live a fulfilling life!

Foods to Eat and Foods to Avoid

Now that you understand the significance of diet, let's look at the sorts of foods to prioritize and those to restrict for successful type 2 diabetes management:

Foods to Embrace:
1. Non-Starchy Vegetables: These are low in calories, carbohydrates, and sugar yet high in vitamins, minerals, and fiber. Think about leafy greens, broccoli, asparagus, cauliflower, bell peppers, mushrooms, and eggplant.
2. Low-Glycemic Fruits: These foods have little effect on blood sugar levels. Berries, apples, pears, grapefruits, and oranges are great options.
3. Whole Grain: Choose whole grains such as brown rice, quinoa, whole wheat bread, and pasta over processed grains. They deliver long-lasting energy and make you feel fuller for longer.
4. Lean Protein Sources: Choose lean proteins such as grilled chicken, fish, beans, lentils, and tofu. Protein promotes satiety and blood sugar regulation.
5. Healthy Fats: Consume healthy fats such as avocados, nuts, seeds, and olive oil. These improve heart health and create a sense of fullness.

Foods To Limit:

1. Sugary Drinks: Sodas, juices, sweetened coffees, and sports drinks have additional sugars, which cause blood sugar to rise. Choose water, unsweetened tea, or black coffee instead.

2. Refined carbs: White bread, spaghetti, pastries, cookies, and cakes include refined carbs, which quickly convert to sugar and raise blood sugar levels.

3. Starchy veggies: Potatoes, maize, and peas contain more carbs than non-starchy veggies. Consume them in moderation and combine them with protein and healthy fats to delay digestion.

4. Processed Foods: These are generally high in harmful fats, added sugars, and salt. Avoid eating processed meats, frozen dinners, packaged snacks, and rapid meals.

5. Unhealthy Fats: Limit the amount of saturated and trans fats in fried meals, fatty meats, and processed snacks. These lead to cardiovascular disease and other health issues.

Eating Out Following Type 2 Diabetes Diet

Eating out does not have to interrupt your healthy eating plans! **Here are some pointers to help you make wise decisions while eating out:**

Preparation Is Key:

1. Check out the menu online (if available): To prevent making impulsive selections, plan your lunch ahead of time.

2. Choose alternatives that promote lean protein, non-starchy veggies, and healthy grains.

3. Consider Portion Sizes: Restaurant servings are often bigger than suggested. Be considerate and share a meal or request a half-portion.

Make Healthy Choices:

1. Pick Grilled, Baked, or Broiled Options: These cooking techniques are healthier than fried or sautéed foods.
2. Ask About Preparations: Inquire about cooking techniques and ingredients. Choose foods with little added sweeteners and sauces on the side.
3. Embrace Salads: Salads make an excellent beginning or light main dish. Choose grilled protein and a mild vinaigrette dressing.
4. Beware of Hidden Sugars: Salad dressings, marinades, and sauces may be high in sugar. Ask for dressings on the side and keep them mild.
5. Fiber Is Your Friend: Choose foods with whole grains or beans for more fiber, which improves fullness and helps manage blood sugar levels.

Mindful Swaps:

1. Substitute Whole Grains for Refined Grains: Replace white rice with brown rice, whole-wheat pasta with regular pasta, or skip bread altogether.
2. Steam or Roast Vegetables Over Fries: Opt for steamed or roasted vegetables instead of french fries or onion rings.
3. Healthy Fat Choices: Opt for olive oil-based dressings instead of creamy ones.

Do Not Forget Beverages:

1. Water is the best choice for staying hydrated and is sugar-free.

2. Unsweetened tea or coffee are healthy alternatives to sugary beverages.

3. Limit alcohol consumption: Alcohol consumption may affect blood sugar levels. If you decide to drink, do so in moderation.

With a little forethought and these guidelines, you can confidently browse restaurant menus and enjoy tasty meals that help you manage type 2 diabetes.

Type 2 Diabetes Shopping List

This shopping list serves as a basis for preparing nutritious meals that will help you manage your type 2 diabetes.

Pantry Staples:

1. Non-Starchy Vegetables: Broccoli, cauliflower, spinach, kale, asparagus, mushrooms, bell peppers, zucchini, eggplant

2. Low-Glycemic Fruits: Berries (fresh or frozen), apples, pears, grapefruits, oranges

3. Whole Grains: Brown rice, quinoa, whole-wheat pasta, whole-wheat bread, oats

4. Lean Protein Sources: Skinless, boneless chicken breasts, fish filets (salmon, tuna, etc.), lean ground turkey, beans (black beans, kidney beans, lentils), tofu

5. Healthy Fats: Olive oil, avocado oil, nuts (almonds, walnuts), nut butters (unsweetened peanut butter, almond butter), seeds (chia seeds, flax seeds)

6. Vinegars: Apple cider vinegar, balsamic vinegar

7. Spices and Herbs: Garlic powder, onion powder, dried oregano, basil, thyme, cinnamon

Fresh Produce:

1. Seasonal Veggies: Choose a range of bright veggies each week.

2. Salad Greens: Mix in your favorite greens, such as romaine, spinach, arugula, or kale.

3. Fruits with Low Sugar Content: Fresh berries are an excellent alternative. Consider other seasonal fruits, such as apples, pears, or grapefruits, in moderation.

Protein Sources:

1. Lean Meats and Poultry: Ground turkey, chicken breasts, or thighs. Choose lean cuts and reduce any apparent fat.

2. Seafood: Choose omega-3-rich seafood such as salmon, tuna, and sardines.

3. Eggs: A flexible protein source for breakfast, lunch, or dinner.

4. Plant-Based Proteins: Tofu, tempeh, lentils, and beans are vegetarian protein sources.

Dairy is Optional:

1. Unsweetened Greek Yogurt: A protein and calcium-rich food. Choose simple variations and add your fruits or flavors.

2. Low-Fat Cottage Cheese: Another source of protein and calcium, ideal for breakfast or snacking.

3. Unsweetened Almond Milk or Other Unsweetened Plant-Based Milk Alternatives: For individuals who are lactose intolerant or eat vegan.

Healthy Fats:

1. Avocados: Rich in healthy fats and fiber.
2. Nuts and Seeds: Almonds, walnuts, chia seeds, and flax seeds are ideal for snacking or adding to salads and yogurt.
3. Olive Oil: Can be used for cooking, salad dressings, or marinades.

Sweeteners (Used sparingly):

1. Sugar substitutes: Choose diabetic-approved replacements, such as stevia or erythritol.

Note:

1. Read the Food Labels: Consider sugar content and pick lower-carbohydrate products.
2. Frozen Options: Frozen fruits and veggies are a practical and cost-effective option.
3. Fresh vs. Canned: Use fresh vegetables wherever feasible. When buying canned foods, aim for those that are packed in water or have a low salt content.
4. Whole Grains versus Refined Grains: For long-term energy and fiber, choose whole grains such as brown rice, quinoa, and whole-wheat bread.

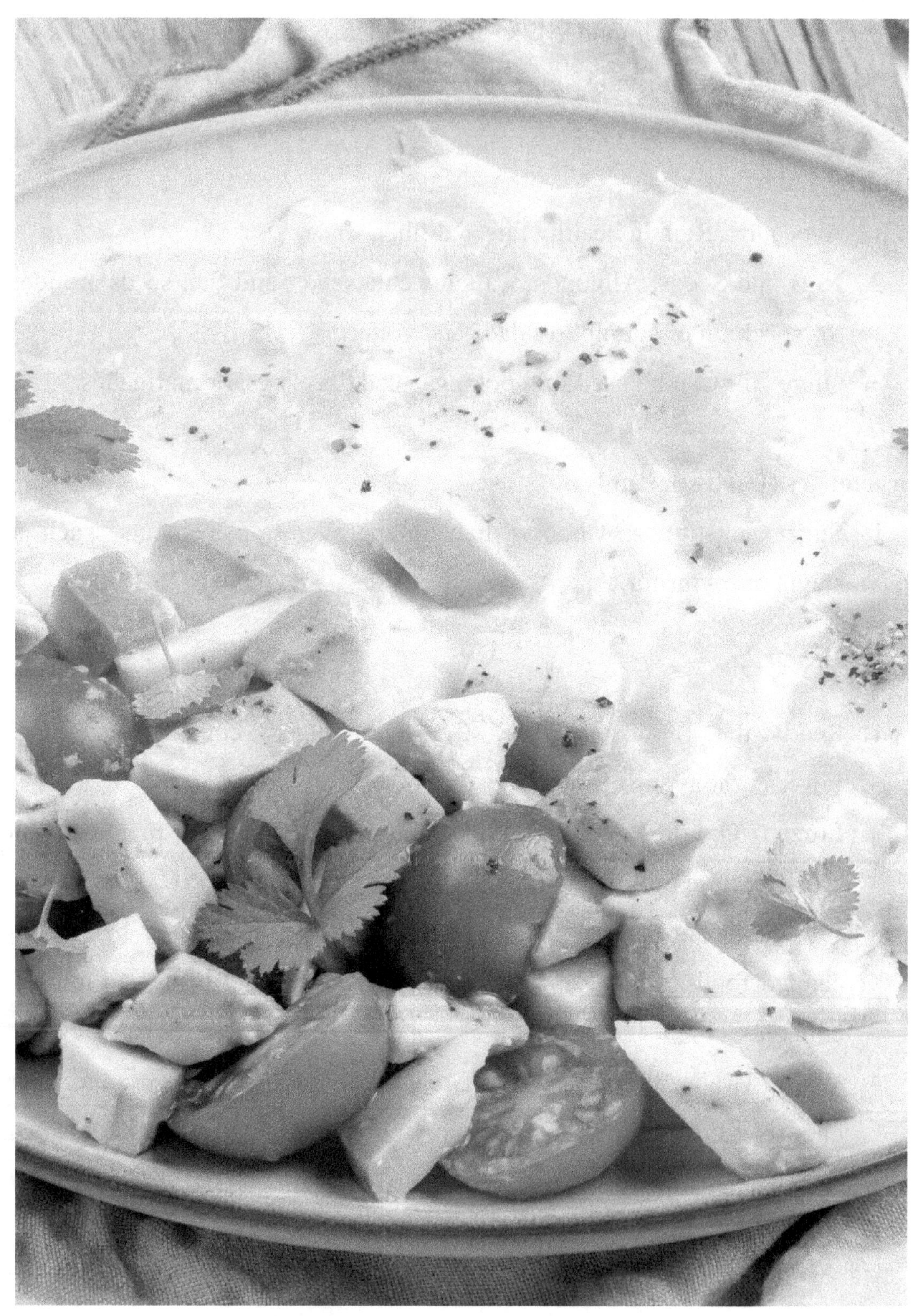

Chapter 3: 42-Day Meal Plan

Day: 1

Breakfast: Smoked Salmon and Veggie Frittata

Lunch: Mediterranean Tuna Salad Pita Pockets

Snack: Edamame Pods with Chili Flakes and Lime

Dinner: Salmon with Lemon Dill Sauce and Roasted Asparagus

Day: 2

Breakfast: Chia Seed Pudding with Berries and Nuts

Lunch: Chicken and Black Bean Salad with Avocado

Snack: Cucumber Slices with Cottage Cheese and Dill

Dinner: Chicken Stir-Fry with Brown Rice and Vegetables

Day: 3

Breakfast: Whole-Wheat Pancakes with Greek Yogurt and Berries

Lunch: Lentil Soup with Whole-Wheat Bread

Snack: Roasted Chickpeas with Rosemary and Garlic

Dinner: Turkey Taco Bowls with Low-Carb Tortillas or Lettuce Wraps

Day: 4

Breakfast: Scrambled Eggs with Avocado and Tomatoes

Lunch: Quinoa Veggie Bowl with Tahini Dressing

Snack: Apple Slices with Almond Butter and Cinnamon

Dinner: One-Pan Lemon Garlic Shrimp with Roasted Vegetables

Day: 5

Breakfast: Spiced Tofu Scramble with Whole-Wheat Toast

Lunch: Salmon with Roasted Asparagus and Quinoa

Snack: Bell Pepper Strips with Guacamole

Dinner: Lentil Shepherd's Pie with Mashed Cauliflower

Day: 6

Breakfast: Overnight Oats with Nut Butter and Sliced Almonds

Lunch: Turkey and Veggie Wraps

Snack: Greek Yogurt with Berries and Chia Seeds

Dinner: Black Bean Burgers on Whole-Wheat Buns with Sweet Potato Fries

Day: 7

Breakfast: Greek Yogurt Parfait with Berries and Granola

Lunch: Open-Faced Egg Salad with Whole-Wheat Toast

Snack: Sliced Pear with a dollop of Ricotta Cheese and a drizzle of Honey

Dinner: Baked Chicken Fajitas with Whole-Wheat Tortillas and Grilled Vegetables

Day: 8

Breakfast: Breakfast Burrito Bowl

Lunch: Chicken Caesar Salad with Light Dressing

Snack: Turkey Roll-Ups with Mustard and Lettuce Wraps

Dinner: Salmon with Roasted Brussels Sprouts and Quinoa

Day: 9

Breakfast: Egg Muffins with Spinach and Feta Cheese

Lunch: Chickpea Salad Sandwich on Whole-Wheat Bread

Snack: Carrot Sticks with Hummus

Dinner: Chicken and Vegetable Curry with Brown Rice

Day: 10

Breakfast: Smoothie with Spinach, Banana, and Almond Milk

Lunch: Black Bean Burgers with Sweet Potato Fries

Snack: Roasted Pumpkin Seeds

Dinner: Tofu Scramble with Whole-Wheat Toast and Avocado

Day: 11

Breakfast: Sweet Potato Toast with Sliced Turkey and Avocado

Lunch: Tuna Poke Bowl with Brown Rice and Edamame

Snack: Seaweed Snacks

Dinner: Tuna Noodle Casserole with Whole-Wheat Noodles and Light Cream Sauce

Day: 12

Breakfast: Breakfast Quesadillas with Whole-Wheat Tortillas

Lunch: Turkey Chili with a Dollop of Greek Yogurt

Snack: Air-Popped Popcorn with Nutritional Yeast

Dinner: Chicken Souvlaki Bowls with Lemon Herb Marinade and Whole-Wheat Pita Bread

Day: 13

Breakfast: High-Protein Pancakes with Cottage Cheese

Lunch: Shrimp Scampi with Zucchini Noodles

Snack: Sliced Bell Peppers with cottage cheese

Dinner: Vegetarian Chili with Kidney Beans and Corn

Day: 14

Breakfast: Baked Oatmeal with Berries and Pecans

Lunch: Chicken and Vegetable Skewers with Peanut Sauce

Snack: Sugar-Snap Peas with a dollop of Peanut Butter

Dinner: Baked Cod with Lemon and Herbs and Roasted Vegetables

Day: 15

Breakfast: Turkey Sausage and Veggie Scramble with Whole-Wheat Toast

Lunch: Lentil and Veggie Stuffed Peppers

Snack: Bell Pepper Strips with Guacamole

Dinner: Chicken and Vegetable Sheet-Pan Dinner

Day: 16

Breakfast: Smoked Salmon and Veggie Frittata

Lunch: Mediterranean Tuna Salad Pita Pockets

Snack: Edamame Pods with Chili Flakes and Lime

Dinner: Salmon with Lemon Dill Sauce and Roasted Asparagus

Day: 17

Breakfast: Chia Seed Pudding with Berries and Nuts

Lunch: Chicken and Black Bean Salad with Avocado

Snack: Cucumber Slices with Cottage Cheese and Dill

Dinner: Chicken Stir-Fry with Brown Rice and Vegetables

Day: 18

Breakfast: Whole-Wheat Pancakes with Greek Yogurt and Berries

Lunch: Lentil Soup with Whole-Wheat Bread

Snack: Roasted Chickpeas with Rosemary and Garlic

Dinner: Turkey Taco Bowls with Low-Carb Tortillas or Lettuce Wraps

Day: 19

Breakfast: Scrambled Eggs with Avocado and Tomatoes

Lunch: Quinoa Veggie Bowl with Tahini Dressing

Snack: Apple Slices with Almond Butter and Cinnamon

Dinner: One-Pan Lemon Garlic Shrimp with Roasted Vegetables

Day: 20

Breakfast: Spiced Tofu Scramble with Whole-Wheat Toast

Lunch: Salmon with Roasted Asparagus and Quinoa

Snack: Bell Pepper Strips with Guacamole

Dinner: Lentil Shepherd's Pie with Mashed Cauliflower

Day: 21

Breakfast: Overnight Oats with Nut Butter and Sliced Almonds

Lunch: Turkey and Veggie Wraps

Snack: Greek Yogurt with Berries and Chia Seeds

Dinner: Black Bean Burgers on Whole-Wheat Buns with Sweet Potato Fries

Day: 22

Breakfast: Greek Yogurt Parfait with Berries and Granola

Lunch: Open-Faced Egg Salad with Whole-Wheat Toast

Snack: Sliced Pear with a dollop of Ricotta Cheese and a drizzle of Honey

Dinner: Baked Chicken Fajitas with Whole-Wheat Tortillas and Grilled Vegetables

Day: 23

Breakfast: Breakfast Burrito Bowl

Lunch: Chicken Caesar Salad with Light Dressing

Snack: Turkey Roll-Ups with Mustard and Lettuce Wraps

Dinner: Salmon with Roasted Brussels Sprouts and Quinoa

Day: 24

Breakfast: Egg Muffins with Spinach and Feta Cheese

Lunch: Chickpea Salad Sandwich on Whole-Wheat Bread

Snack: Carrot Sticks with Hummus

Dinner: Chicken and Vegetable Curry with Brown Rice

Day: 25

Breakfast: Smoothie with Spinach, Banana, and Almond Milk

Lunch: Black Bean Burgers with Sweet Potato Fries

Snack: Roasted Pumpkin Seeds

Dinner: Tofu Scramble with Whole-Wheat Toast and Avocado

Day: 26

Breakfast: Sweet Potato Toast with Sliced Turkey and Avocado

Lunch: Tuna Poke Bowl with Brown Rice and Edamame

Snack: Seaweed Snacks

Dinner: Tuna Noodle Casserole with Whole-Wheat Noodles and Light Cream Sauce

Day: 27

Breakfast: Breakfast Quesadillas with Whole-Wheat Tortillas

Lunch: Turkey Chili with a Dollop of Greek Yogurt

Snack: Air-Popped Popcorn with Nutritional Yeast

Dinner: Chicken Souvlaki Bowls with Lemon Herb Marinade and Whole-Wheat Pita Bread

Day: 28

Breakfast: High-Protein Pancakes with Cottage Cheese

Lunch: Shrimp Scampi with Zucchini Noodles

Snack: Sliced Bell Peppers with cottage cheese

Dinner: Vegetarian Chili with Kidney Beans and Corn

Day: 29

Breakfast: Baked Oatmeal with Berries and Pecans

Lunch: Chicken and Vegetable Skewers with Peanut Sauce

Snack: Sugar-Snap Peas with a dollop of Peanut Butter

Dinner: Baked Cod with Lemon and Herbs and Roasted Vegetables

Day: 30

Breakfast: Turkey Sausage and Veggie Scramble with Whole-Wheat Toast

Lunch: Lentil and Veggie Stuffed Peppers

Snack: Bell Pepper Strips with Guacamole

Dinner: Chicken and Vegetable Sheet-Pan Dinner

Day: 31

Breakfast: Smoked Salmon and Veggie Frittata

Lunch: Mediterranean Tuna Salad Pita Pockets

Snack: Edamame Pods with Chili Flakes and Lime

Dinner: Salmon with Lemon Dill Sauce and Roasted Asparagus

Day: 32

Breakfast: Chia Seed Pudding with Berries and Nuts

Lunch: Chicken and Black Bean Salad with Avocado

Snack: Cucumber Slices with Cottage Cheese and Dill

Dinner: Chicken Stir-Fry with Brown Rice and Vegetables

Day: 33

Breakfast: Whole-Wheat Pancakes with Greek Yogurt and Berries

Lunch: Lentil Soup with Whole-Wheat Bread

Snack: Roasted Chickpeas with Rosemary and Garlic

Dinner: Turkey Taco Bowls with Low-Carb Tortillas or Lettuce Wraps

Day: 34

Breakfast: Scrambled Eggs with Avocado and Tomatoes

Lunch: Quinoa Veggie Bowl with Tahini Dressing

Snack: Apple Slices with Almond Butter and Cinnamon

Dinner: One-Pan Lemon Garlic Shrimp with Roasted Vegetables

Day: 35

Breakfast: Spiced Tofu Scramble with Whole-Wheat Toast

Lunch: Salmon with Roasted Asparagus and Quinoa

Snack: Bell Pepper Strips with Guacamole

Dinner: Lentil Shepherd's Pie with Mashed Cauliflower

Day: 36

Breakfast: Overnight Oats with Nut Butter and Sliced Almonds

Lunch: Turkey and Veggie Wraps

Snack: Greek Yogurt with Berries and Chia Seeds

Dinner: Black Bean Burgers on Whole-Wheat Buns with Sweet Potato Fries

Day: 37

Breakfast: Greek Yogurt Parfait with Berries and Granola

Lunch: Open-Faced Egg Salad with Whole-Wheat Toast

Snack: Sliced Pear with a dollop of Ricotta Cheese and a drizzle of Honey

Dinner: Baked Chicken Fajitas with Whole-Wheat Tortillas and Grilled Vegetables

Day: 38

Breakfast: Breakfast Burrito Bowl

Lunch: Chicken Caesar Salad with Light Dressing

Snack: Turkey Roll-Ups with Mustard and Lettuce Wraps

Dinner: Salmon with Roasted Brussels Sprouts and Quinoa

Breakfast: Egg Muffins with Spinach and Feta Cheese

Lunch: Chickpea Salad Sandwich on Whole-Wheat Bread

Snack: Carrot Sticks with Hummus

Dinner: Chicken and Vegetable Curry with Brown Rice

Breakfast: Smoothie with Spinach, Banana, and Almond Milk

Lunch: Black Bean Burgers with Sweet Potato Fries

Snack: Roasted Pumpkin Seeds

Dinner: Tofu Scramble with Whole-Wheat Toast and Avocado

Breakfast: Sweet Potato Toast with Sliced Turkey and Avocado

Lunch: Tuna Poke Bowl with Brown Rice and Edamame

Snack: Seaweed Snacks

Dinner: Tuna Noodle Casserole with Whole-Wheat Noodles and Light Cream Sauce

Breakfast: Breakfast Quesadillas with Whole-Wheat Tortillas

Lunch: Turkey Chili with a Dollop of Greek Yogurt

Snack: Air-Popped Popcorn with Nutritional Yeast

Dinner: Chicken Souvlaki Bowls with Lemon Herb Marinade and Whole-Wheat Pita Bread

Chapter 4: Breakfast Recipes

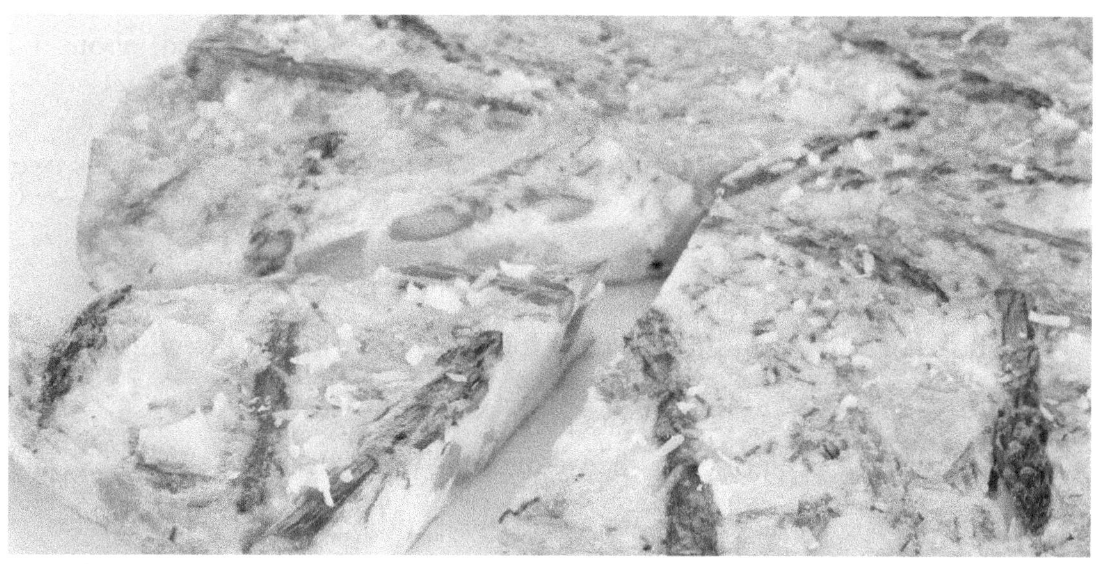

Smoked Salmon and Veggie Frittata

Ingredients:

- 4 large eggs
- 1/4 cup diced red bell pepper
- 1/4 cup diced onion
- 1/4 cup chopped spinach
- 2 ounces smoked salmon, chopped
- 1 tablespoon olive oil
- Salt and pepper to taste
- 2 tablespoons grated Parmesan cheese (optional)

Directions:

1. Preheat your oven to 350°F (175°C).
2. In a mixing bowl, whisk the eggs until well beaten. Season with salt and pepper to taste.
3. Heat olive oil in an oven-safe skillet over medium heat.

4. Add diced red bell pepper and onion to the skillet. Sauté until they are soft, about 3-4 minutes.

5. Add chopped spinach to the skillet and cook until wilted, about 1-2 minutes.

6. Spread the veggies evenly in the skillet and pour the beaten eggs over them.

7. Place chopped smoked salmon evenly on top of the egg mixture.

8. Cook the frittata on the stovetop for 3-4 minutes until the edges start to set.

9. Sprinkle grated Parmesan cheese over the top if desired.

10. Transfer the skillet to the preheated oven and bake for 10-12 minutes, or until the frittata is set in the center and lightly golden on top.

11. Once cooked, remove from the oven and let it cool for a few minutes.

12. Slice the frittata into wedges and serve warm.

Chia Seed Pudding with Berries and Nuts

Ingredients:

- 1/4 cup chia seeds
- 1 cup unsweetened almond milk (or any milk of your choice)
- 1/2 teaspoon vanilla extract
- 1 tablespoon honey or maple syrup (optional)
- 1/4 cup mixed berries (such as strawberries, blueberries, or raspberries)
- 2 tablespoons chopped nuts (such as almonds, walnuts, or pecans)

Directions:

1. In a mixing bowl or jar, combine chia seeds, unsweetened almond milk, vanilla extract, and honey or maple syrup if using. Stir well to combine.

2. Cover the bowl or jar and refrigerate for at least 2 hours or overnight, allowing the chia seeds to absorb the liquid and thicken into a pudding-like consistency.

3. After the pudding has set, give it a good stir to ensure that the chia seeds are evenly distributed.

4. Divide the chia seed pudding into serving bowls or glasses.

5. Top each serving with mixed berries and chopped nuts.

6. Serve immediately, or store in the refrigerator for up to 3 days.

Whole-Wheat Pancakes with Greek Yogurt and Berries

Ingredients:

- 1 cup whole wheat flour
- 1 tablespoon baking powder
- 1/4 teaspoon salt
- 1 tablespoon honey or maple syrup
- 1 cup unsweetened almond milk (or any milk of your choice)
- 1 large egg
- 1 tablespoon olive oil or melted coconut oil
- 1/2 teaspoon vanilla extract
- Cooking spray or additional oil for greasing the pan
- 1/2 cup plain Greek yogurt
- 1/2 cup mixed berries (such as strawberries, blueberries, or raspberries)

Directions:

1. In a large mixing bowl, whisk together the whole wheat flour, baking powder, and salt.

2. In a separate bowl, whisk together the honey or maple syrup, almond milk, egg, olive oil, and vanilla extract until well combined.

3. Pour the wet ingredients into the dry ingredients and stir until just combined. Do not overmix; a few lumps are okay.

4. Heat a non-stick skillet or griddle over medium heat and lightly grease with cooking spray or a small amount of oil.

5. Pour 1/4 cup of the pancake batter onto the skillet for each pancake.

6. Cook until bubbles form on the surface of the pancakes and the edges look set, about 2-3 minutes.

7. Flip the pancakes and cook for an additional 1-2 minutes, until golden brown and cooked through.

8. Remove the pancakes from the skillet and repeat with the remaining batter.

9. To serve, top each pancake with a dollop of Greek yogurt and a handful of mixed berries.

10. Optional: Drizzle with a little honey or maple syrup for added sweetness.

Scrambled Eggs with Avocado and Tomatoes

Ingredients:

- 2 large eggs
- 1/2 ripe avocado, diced
- 1/2 cup cherry tomatoes, halved
- 1 tablespoon olive oil
- Salt and pepper to taste
- Optional: chopped fresh herbs such as parsley or cilantro for garnish

Directions:

1. In a small bowl, whisk the eggs together until well beaten. Season with salt and pepper to taste.
2. Heat olive oil in a non-stick skillet over medium heat.
3. Add the diced avocado to the skillet and cook for 1-2 minutes, stirring occasionally until slightly softened.
4. Add the halved cherry tomatoes to the skillet and cook for an additional 1-2 minutes until they start to soften.
5. Pour the beaten eggs into the skillet with the avocado and tomatoes.
6. Using a spatula, gently scramble the eggs, stirring occasionally, until they are cooked to your desired consistency.
7. Once the eggs are cooked, remove the skillet from the heat.
8. Serve the scrambled eggs with avocado and tomatoes hot, garnished with chopped fresh herbs if desired.

Spiced Tofu Scramble with Whole-Wheat Toast

Ingredients:

- 1/2 block (about 7 oz) firm tofu, drained and crumbled
- 1/4 cup diced bell peppers (any color)
- 1/4 cup diced onion
- 1/4 cup chopped spinach
- 1 clove garlic, minced
- 1/2 teaspoon ground turmeric
- 1/4 teaspoon ground cumin
- 1/4 teaspoon paprika
- Salt and pepper to taste
- 1 tablespoon olive oil

- 2 slices whole-wheat bread, toasted

- Optional toppings: sliced avocado, salsa, hot sauce

Directions:

1. Heat olive oil in a non-stick skillet over medium heat.

2. Add diced bell peppers and onions to the skillet. Sauté until they are soft, about 3-4 minutes.

3. Add minced garlic to the skillet and cook for an additional 1 minute until fragrant.

4. Add crumbled tofu to the skillet along with ground turmeric, ground cumin, paprika, salt, and pepper. Stir well to combine.

5. Cook the tofu mixture for 5-6 minutes, stirring occasionally, until the tofu is heated through and lightly browned.

6. Add chopped spinach to the skillet and cook for another 1-2 minutes until wilted.

7. While the tofu scramble is cooking, toast the whole-wheat bread slices until golden brown.

8. Serve the spiced tofu scramble hot with whole-wheat toast on the side.

9. Optional: Top the tofu scramble with sliced avocado, salsa, or hot sauce for extra flavor.

Overnight Oats with Nut Butter and Sliced Almonds

Ingredients:

- 1/2 cup rolled oats (old-fashioned oats)

- 1/2 cup unsweetened almond milk (or any milk of your choice)

- 1 tablespoon nut butter (such as almond butter or peanut butter)

- 1 tablespoon sliced almonds

- 1/2 teaspoon ground cinnamon
- 1/2 teaspoon vanilla extract
- Optional: 1 teaspoon honey or maple syrup for sweetness
- Optional toppings: fresh berries, banana slices, additional nut butter

Directions:

1. In a mason jar or airtight container, combine rolled oats, almond milk, nut butter, sliced almonds, ground cinnamon, and vanilla extract. If desired, add honey or maple syrup for sweetness.
2. Stir well to combine all the ingredients.
3. Cover the jar or container with a lid and refrigerate overnight, or for at least 4 hours, to allow the oats to soften and absorb the liquid.
4. In the morning, give the overnight oats a good stir.
5. If the consistency is too thick, you can add a splash of almond milk to loosen it up.
6. Serve the overnight oats cold, topped with additional nut butter, fresh berries, banana slices, or any other toppings of your choice.

Greek Yogurt Parfait with Berries and Granola

Ingredients:

- 1/2 cup plain Greek yogurt
- 1/4 cup mixed berries (such as strawberries, blueberries, or raspberries)
- 2 tablespoons granola (choose a low-sugar or sugar-free option)
- Optional: 1 teaspoon honey or maple syrup for added sweetness

Directions:

1. In a serving glass or bowl, layer half of the Greek yogurt.
2. Add half of the mixed berries on top of the yogurt layer.
3. Sprinkle one tablespoon of granola over the berries.

4. Repeat the layers with the remaining yogurt, berries, and granola.

5. Drizzle with honey or maple syrup if desired for added sweetness.

6. Serve immediately and enjoy!

Breakfast Burrito Bowl

Ingredients:

- 1/2 cup cooked quinoa or brown rice
- 2 large eggs
- 1/4 cup black beans, rinsed and drained
- 1/4 cup diced bell peppers (any color)
- 1/4 cup diced onion
- 1/4 cup salsa
- 1/4 avocado, sliced
- 1 tablespoon chopped cilantro (optional)
- Salt and pepper to taste
- Cooking spray or olive oil for cooking

Directions:

1. Heat a non-stick skillet over medium heat and lightly coat with cooking spray or olive oil.

2. Crack the eggs into the skillet and cook them to your desired style (scrambled, fried, or poached). Season with salt and pepper to taste.

3. While the eggs are cooking, heat the black beans in a small saucepan or in the microwave until warmed through.

4. In the same skillet used for the eggs, add diced bell peppers and onions. Sauté until they are soft, about 3-4 minutes.

5. To assemble the burrito bowl, start with a base of cooked quinoa or brown rice in a bowl.

6. Top with the cooked eggs, sautéed bell peppers and onions, and warmed black beans.

7. Drizzle salsa over the top of the bowl.

8. Garnish with sliced avocado and chopped cilantro, if desired.

9. Serve hot and enjoy!

Egg Muffins with Spinach and Feta Cheese

Ingredients:

- 6 large eggs
- 1 cup fresh spinach, chopped
- 1/4 cup crumbled feta cheese
- 1/4 cup diced bell peppers (any color)
- 1/4 cup diced onion
- 1 tablespoon olive oil
- Salt and pepper to taste
- Cooking spray or olive oil for greasing the muffin tin

Directions:

1. Preheat your oven to 350°F (175°C) and grease a muffin tin with cooking spray or olive oil.

2. Heat olive oil in a skillet over medium heat.

3. Add diced bell peppers and onions to the skillet. Sauté until they are soft, about 3-4 minutes.

4. Add chopped spinach to the skillet and cook until wilted, about 1-2 minutes.

5. In a mixing bowl, beat the eggs until well combined. Season with salt and pepper to taste.

6. Stir in the sautéed vegetables and crumbled feta cheese into the beaten eggs.

7. Pour the egg mixture evenly into the prepared muffin tin, filling each cup about 3/4 full.

8. Bake in the preheated oven for 20-25 minutes, or until the egg muffins are set in the center and lightly golden on top.

9. Remove from the oven and let the egg muffins cool in the muffin tin for a few minutes before carefully removing them.

10. Serve warm or at room temperature.

Smoothie with Spinach, Banana, and Almond Milk

Ingredients:

- 1 ripe banana, peeled and sliced
- 1 cup fresh spinach leaves
- 1/2 cup unsweetened almond milk (or any milk of your choice)
- 1/4 cup plain Greek yogurt (optional, for added creaminess)
- 1 tablespoon almond butter (or peanut butter)
- 1/2 teaspoon honey or maple syrup (optional, for added sweetness)
- Ice cubes (optional, for a colder smoothie)

Directions:

1. Place all the ingredients in a blender.

2. Blend until smooth and creamy, adding more almond milk if needed to reach your desired consistency.

3. Taste and adjust sweetness, if necessary, by adding honey or maple syrup.

4. If you prefer a colder smoothie, add a few ice cubes and blend again until smooth.

5. Pour the smoothie into a glass and serve immediately.

Sweet Potato Toast with Sliced Turkey and Avocado

Ingredients:

- 1 medium sweet potato
- 2 slices of cooked turkey breast
- 1/2 avocado, sliced
- Salt and pepper to taste
- Optional toppings: sliced tomato, sprouts, mustard or hummus

Directions:

1. Wash the sweet potato thoroughly and slice it lengthwise into 1/4 inch thick slices.

2. Place the sweet potato slices in a toaster and toast until they are cooked through and tender. You may need to toast them multiple times depending on the thickness of the slices and the power of your toaster.

3. Once the sweet potato slices are toasted, remove them from the toaster and let them cool slightly.

4. Top each sweet potato slice with a slice of cooked turkey breast.

5. Add sliced avocado on top of the turkey.

6. Season with salt and pepper to taste.

7. If desired, add additional toppings such as sliced tomato, sprouts, mustard, or hummus for extra flavor and nutrition.

8. Serve immediately and enjoy!

Breakfast Quesadillas with Whole-Wheat Tortillas

Ingredients:

- 2 whole wheat tortillas
- 2 large eggs
- 1/4 cup shredded cheese (cheddar, mozzarella, or your choice)
- 1/4 cup diced bell peppers (any color)
- 1/4 cup diced onion
- 2 slices cooked turkey bacon or ham (optional)
- Salt and pepper to taste
- Cooking spray or olive oil for cooking

Directions:

1. In a non-stick skillet, cook the diced bell peppers and onions over medium heat until they are soft, about 3-4 minutes. If using turkey bacon or ham, cook it in the skillet until crispy, then remove and set aside.
2. In the same skillet, crack the eggs and cook them to your desired style (scrambled, fried, or poached). Season with salt and pepper to taste.
3. Once the eggs are cooked, remove them from the skillet and set aside.
4. Wipe the skillet clean and return it to the heat. Lightly coat with cooking spray or olive oil.
5. Place one whole wheat tortilla in the skillet. Sprinkle half of the shredded cheese evenly over the tortilla.
6. Arrange the cooked eggs, cooked bell peppers and onions, and turkey bacon or ham (if using) on top of the cheese.
7. Sprinkle the remaining shredded cheese over the filling ingredients.
8. Top with the second whole wheat tortilla.

9. Cook the quesadilla for 2-3 minutes on each side, or until the tortillas are golden brown and the cheese is melted.

10. Once cooked, remove the quesadilla from the skillet and let it cool for a minute before slicing into wedges.

11. Serve hot and enjoy!

High-Protein Pancakes with Cottage Cheese

Ingredients:

- 1/2 cup rolled oats
- 1/2 cup cottage cheese
- 2 large eggs
- 1 tablespoon honey or maple syrup (optional)
- 1/2 teaspoon vanilla extract
- 1/2 teaspoon baking powder
- Cooking spray or olive oil for cooking

Directions:

1. In a blender or food processor, combine rolled oats, cottage cheese, eggs, honey or maple syrup (if using), vanilla extract, and baking powder.

2. Blend until smooth and well combined. The batter should have a smooth consistency.

3. Heat a non-stick skillet or griddle over medium heat. Lightly coat with cooking spray or olive oil.

4. Pour about 1/4 cup of the pancake batter onto the skillet for each pancake.

5. Cook until bubbles form on the surface of the pancakes and the edges look set, about 2-3 minutes.

6. Flip the pancakes and cook for an additional 1-2 minutes, until golden brown and cooked through.

7. Remove the pancakes from the skillet and repeat with the remaining batter.

8. Serve the pancakes warm, topped with your favorite toppings such as fresh berries, sliced banana, Greek yogurt, or a drizzle of honey.

Baked Oatmeal with Berries and Pecans

Ingredients:

- 2 cups old-fashioned oats
- 1 teaspoon baking powder
- 1/2 teaspoon ground cinnamon
- 1/4 teaspoon salt
- 2 cups unsweetened almond milk (or any milk of your choice)
- 1/4 cup pure maple syrup or honey
- 1 large egg
- 2 tablespoons melted coconut oil or butter
- 1 teaspoon vanilla extract
- 1 cup mixed berries (such as blueberries, strawberries, raspberries)
- 1/4 cup chopped pecans (or any nuts of your choice)
- Optional toppings: additional berries, Greek yogurt, or a drizzle of maple syrup

Directions:

1. Preheat your oven to 375°F (190°C). Grease a 9x9 inch baking dish with cooking spray or oil.

2. In a large mixing bowl, combine the oats, baking powder, ground cinnamon, and salt.

3. In another bowl, whisk together the almond milk, maple syrup or honey, egg, melted coconut oil or butter, and vanilla extract until well combined.

4. Pour the wet ingredients into the bowl with the dry ingredients and stir until everything is evenly combined.

5. Gently fold in the mixed berries and chopped pecans.

6. Pour the mixture into the prepared baking dish and spread it out evenly.

7. Bake in the preheated oven for 35-40 minutes, or until the top is golden brown and the oatmeal is set.

8. Remove from the oven and let it cool for a few minutes before slicing and serving.

9. Serve warm, topped with additional berries, Greek yogurt, or a drizzle of maple syrup if desired.

Turkey Sausage and Veggie Scramble with Whole-Wheat Toast

Ingredients:

- 2 whole-wheat bread slices, toasted
- 2 large eggs
- 2 turkey sausage patties, crumbled
- 1/4 cup diced bell peppers (any color)
- 1/4 cup diced onion
- 1/4 cup chopped spinach
- 1 tablespoon olive oil
- Salt and pepper to taste
- Optional toppings: sliced avocado, salsa, hot sauce

Directions:

1. Heat olive oil in a skillet over medium heat.
2. Add diced bell peppers and onions to the skillet. Sauté until they are soft, about 3-4 minutes.
3. Add crumbled turkey sausage patties to the skillet and cook until they are browned and cooked through.
4. Add chopped spinach to the skillet and cook until wilted, about 1-2 minutes.
5. In a bowl, beat the eggs with salt and pepper to taste.
6. Pour the beaten eggs into the skillet with the sausage and veggies.
7. Gently scramble the eggs with the sausage and veggies until cooked to your desired consistency.
8. Once cooked, remove the skillet from the heat.
9. Serve the turkey sausage and veggie scramble hot with whole-wheat toast on the side.
10. Optional: Top the scramble with sliced avocado, salsa, or hot sauce for extra flavor.

Yogurt Bowl with Granola and Pumpkin Seeds

Ingredients:

- 1/2 cup plain Greek yogurt
- 1/4 cup granola (choose a low-sugar or sugar-free option)
- 1 tablespoon pumpkin seeds
- Optional toppings: sliced strawberries, blueberries, or banana

Directions:

1. In a bowl, scoop out the plain Greek yogurt.
2. Sprinkle granola evenly over the yogurt.

3. Add pumpkin seeds on top of the granola.

4. If desired, add additional toppings such as sliced strawberries, blueberries, or bananas.

5. Enjoy immediately!

Breakfast Salad with Grilled Chicken and Berries

Ingredients:

- 2 cups mixed salad greens (such as spinach, arugula, and romaine lettuce)
- 4 ounces grilled chicken breast, sliced
- 1/2 cup mixed berries (such as strawberries, blueberries, and raspberries)
- 1/4 cup sliced almonds or walnuts
- 1/4 cup crumbled feta or goat cheese
- Balsamic vinaigrette dressing

Directions:

1. In a large bowl, combine the mixed salad greens.

2. Top the greens with sliced grilled chicken breast.

3. Scatter the mixed berries over the salad.

4. Sprinkle sliced almonds or walnuts and crumbled feta or goat cheese on top.

5. Drizzle balsamic vinaigrette dressing over the salad, to taste.

6. Toss the salad gently to combine all the ingredients.

7. Serve immediately and enjoy!

Cacao Overnight Oats with Chia Seeds and Almonds

Ingredients:

- 1/2 cup rolled oats
- 1 tablespoon chia seeds
- 1 tablespoon unsweetened cacao powder
- 1 tablespoon maple syrup or honey (optional)
- 1/2 cup unsweetened almond milk (or any milk of your choice)
- 1/4 teaspoon vanilla extract
- 2 tablespoons sliced almonds

Directions:

1. In a mason jar or airtight container, combine the rolled oats, chia seeds, cacao powder, and maple syrup or honey (if using).
2. Pour in the almond milk and add the vanilla extract.
3. Stir well to combine all the ingredients.
4. Cover the jar or container with a lid and refrigerate overnight, or for at least 4 hours, to allow the oats and chia seeds to absorb the liquid and soften.
5. In the morning, give the overnight oats a good stir.
6. If the consistency is too thick, you can add a splash of almond milk to loosen it up.
7. Top the overnight oats with sliced almonds before serving.
8. Enjoy cold straight from the fridge, or you can heat them up in the microwave if you prefer warm oats.

Chapter 5: Lunch Recipes

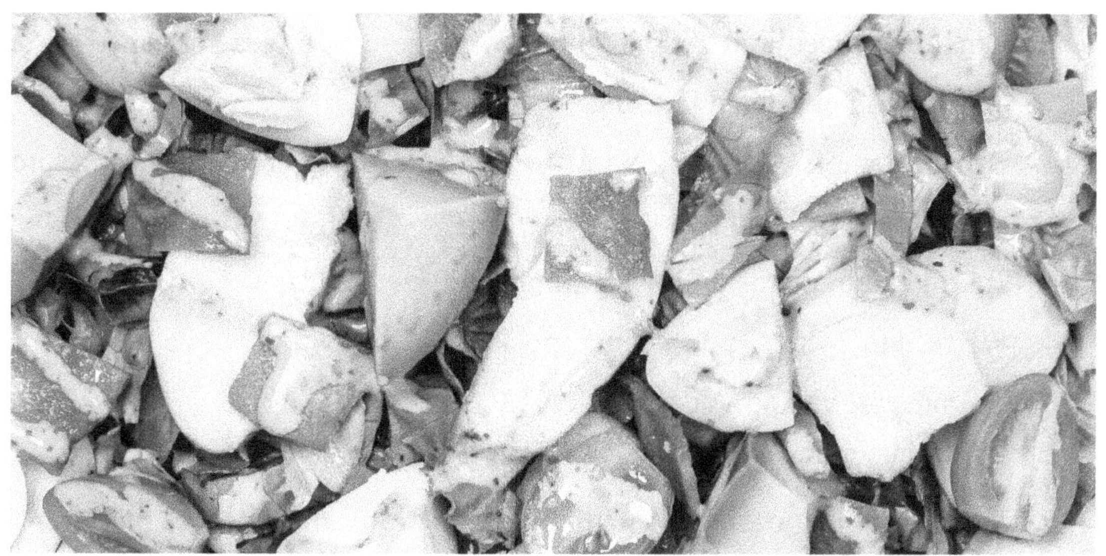

Mediterranean Tuna Salad Pita Pockets

Ingredients:

- 1 can (5 oz) tuna, drained
- 1/4 cup diced cucumber
- 1/4 cup diced tomatoes
- 2 tablespoons diced red onion
- 2 tablespoons chopped Kalamata olives
- 2 tablespoons chopped fresh parsley
- 2 tablespoons crumbled feta cheese
- 1 tablespoon lemon juice
- 1 tablespoon extra virgin olive oil
- Salt and pepper to taste
- 2 whole wheat pita pockets, halved
- 1 cup mixed salad greens (optional, for serving)

Directions:

1. In a mixing bowl, combine the drained tuna, diced cucumber, diced tomatoes, diced red onion, chopped Kalamata olives, chopped fresh parsley, and crumbled feta cheese.

2. Drizzle lemon juice and extra virgin olive oil over the tuna mixture. Season with salt and pepper to taste.

3. Toss the ingredients until well combined.

4. Warm the whole wheat pita pockets in the microwave for 10-15 seconds, or until soft and pliable.

5. Carefully open each pita pocket half to create a pocket.

6. Stuff each pita pocket half with the Mediterranean tuna salad mixture.

7. Optionally, add a handful of mixed salad greens into each pita pocket for extra freshness and crunch.

8. Serve immediately and enjoy!

Chicken and Black Bean Salad with Avocado

Ingredients:

- 2 cups cooked chicken breast, shredded or diced
- 1 can (15 oz) black beans, rinsed and drained
- 1 avocado, diced
- 1 cup cherry tomatoes, halved
- 1/4 cup diced red onion
- 1/4 cup chopped fresh cilantro
- Juice of 1 lime
- 2 tablespoons extra virgin olive oil
- Salt and pepper to taste

- Optional toppings: sliced jalapeno, diced bell peppers, crumbled feta cheese

Directions:

1. In a large mixing bowl, combine the cooked chicken breast, black beans, diced avocado, cherry tomatoes, diced red onion, and chopped fresh cilantro.
2. In a small bowl, whisk together the lime juice and extra virgin olive oil to make the dressing.
3. Pour the dressing over the chicken and black bean mixture.
4. Season with salt and pepper to taste, and toss gently to coat all the ingredients with the dressing.
5. Serve the salad immediately, or refrigerate for 30 minutes to allow the flavors to meld.
6. Optionally, top the salad with sliced jalapeno, diced bell peppers, or crumbled feta cheese for extra flavor and texture.
7. Enjoy!

Lentil Soup with Whole-Wheat Bread

Ingredients:

- 1 cup dried lentils, rinsed and drained
- 1 onion, chopped
- 2 carrots, diced
- 2 celery stalks, diced
- 2 cloves garlic, minced
- 6 cups vegetable or chicken broth (low-sodium)
- 1 can (14.5 oz) diced tomatoes
- 1 teaspoon ground cumin

- 1 teaspoon ground coriander

- 1/2 teaspoon smoked paprika

- Salt and pepper to taste

- 2 tablespoons olive oil

- Fresh parsley or cilantro for garnish (optional)

- Whole-wheat bread slices, toasted

Directions:

1. In a large pot, heat olive oil over medium heat. Add chopped onion, diced carrots, and diced celery. Cook until vegetables are softened, about 5 minutes.

2. Add minced garlic and cook for another minute until fragrant.

3. Add rinsed lentils, diced tomatoes, vegetable or chicken broth, ground cumin, ground coriander, smoked paprika, salt, and pepper to the pot. Stir to combine.

4. Bring the soup to a boil, then reduce the heat to low and let it simmer, covered, for about 25-30 minutes, or until the lentils are tender.

5. Once the lentils are cooked, taste the soup and adjust seasoning as needed.

6. Serve the lentil soup hot, garnished with fresh parsley or cilantro if desired, and accompanied by toasted whole-wheat bread slices.

Quinoa Veggie Bowl with Tahini Dressing

Ingredients:

For the Quinoa Veggie Bowl:

- 1 cup quinoa, rinsed

- 2 cups water or vegetable broth

- 1 tablespoon olive oil

- 1 red bell pepper, diced

- 1 yellow bell pepper, diced

- 1 zucchini, diced

- 1 cup cherry tomatoes, halved

- 1 cup baby spinach or kale

- Salt and pepper to taste

For the Tahini Dressing:

- 1/4 cup tahini

- 2 tablespoons lemon juice

- 1 tablespoon maple syrup or honey

- 1 clove garlic, minced

- 2-4 tablespoons water, to thin as needed

- Salt and pepper to taste

Optional toppings:

- Toasted sesame seeds

- Chopped fresh parsley or cilantro

- Sliced avocado

Directions:

1. In a medium saucepan, combine the rinsed quinoa and water or vegetable broth. Bring to a boil, then reduce heat to low, cover, and simmer for about 15-20 minutes, or until quinoa is cooked and water is absorbed. Remove from heat and let it sit, covered, for 5 minutes. Fluff with a fork.

2. While the quinoa is cooking, heat olive oil in a large skillet over medium heat. Add diced bell peppers and zucchini. Cook, stirring occasionally, for about 5-7 minutes, or until vegetables are tender.

3. Add cherry tomatoes to the skillet and cook for another 2-3 minutes, until they start to soften.

4. Stir in baby spinach or kale and cook until wilted, about 1-2 minutes. Season with salt and pepper to taste.

5. In a small bowl, whisk together tahini, lemon juice, maple syrup or honey, minced garlic, and water until smooth and creamy. Add more water as needed to reach your desired consistency. Season with salt and pepper to taste.

6. To assemble the bowls, divide cooked quinoa among serving bowls. Top with sautéed vegetables. Drizzle with tahini dressing.

7. Garnish with toasted sesame seeds, chopped fresh parsley or cilantro, and sliced avocado, if desired.

8. Serve immediately and enjoy!

Salmon with Roasted Asparagus and Quinoa

Ingredients:

- 2 salmon filets (about 6 oz each)
- 1 bunch asparagus, trimmed
- 1 tablespoon olive oil
- Salt and pepper to taste
- 1 cup quinoa, rinsed
- 2 cups water or vegetable broth
- 1 lemon, sliced
- Fresh dill or parsley for garnish (optional)

Directions:

1. Preheat your oven to 400°F (200°C).

2. Place the salmon filets on a baking sheet lined with parchment paper or aluminum foil. Season the salmon with salt, pepper, and a drizzle of olive oil. Place a couple of lemon slices on top of each filet.

3. Arrange the trimmed asparagus spears on the same baking sheet, next to the salmon filets. Drizzle with olive oil and season with salt and pepper.

4. Roast the salmon and asparagus in the preheated oven for 12-15 minutes, or until the salmon is cooked through and flakes easily with a fork, and the asparagus is tender.

5. While the salmon and asparagus are roasting, prepare the quinoa. In a medium saucepan, combine the rinsed quinoa and water or vegetable broth. Bring to a boil, then reduce heat to low, cover, and simmer for about 15 minutes, or until quinoa is cooked and water is absorbed. Remove from heat and let it sit, covered, for 5 minutes. Fluff with a fork.

6. To serve, divide cooked quinoa among serving plates. Top with roasted salmon filets and asparagus spears. Garnish with fresh dill or parsley, if desired.

7. Serve immediately and enjoy!

Turkey and Veggie Wraps

Ingredients:

- 4 whole wheat or spinach wraps
- 8 slices of turkey breast
- 1/2 cup hummus
- 1 cup shredded lettuce or mixed greens
- 1/2 cup sliced cucumber
- 1/2 cup sliced bell peppers (any color)

- 1/4 cup sliced red onion
- 1/4 cup shredded carrots
- Salt and pepper to taste
- Optional: sliced avocado, sprouts, shredded cheese

Directions:

1. Lay out the whole wheat or spinach wraps on a clean surface.
2. Spread about 2 tablespoons of hummus evenly on each wrap.
3. Place 2 slices of turkey breast on each wrap, towards one end.
4. Layer shredded lettuce or mixed greens, sliced cucumber, sliced bell peppers, sliced red onion, and shredded carrots on top of the turkey slices.
5. Season with salt and pepper to taste.
6. If desired, add optional toppings such as sliced avocado, sprouts, or shredded cheese.
7. Roll up each wrap tightly, folding in the sides as you go, to form a burrito-like shape.
8. Slice each wrap in half diagonally, if desired, and serve immediately.

Open-Faced Egg Salad with Whole-Wheat Toast

Ingredients:

- 4 hard-boiled eggs, peeled and chopped
- 1/4 cup Greek yogurt or mayonnaise (choose low-fat or light options if desired)
- 1 tablespoon Dijon mustard
- 2 tablespoons chopped chives or green onions
- 1/4 teaspoon garlic powder
- Salt and pepper to taste

- 4 slices whole wheat bread, toasted
- Optional toppings: sliced tomatoes, avocado, lettuce, sprouts

Directions:

1. In a mixing bowl, combine the chopped hard-boiled eggs, Greek yogurt or mayonnaise, Dijon mustard, chopped chives or green onions, garlic powder, salt, and pepper. Mix until well combined.
2. Taste and adjust seasoning if necessary.
3. Place the toasted whole wheat bread slices on a plate.
4. Divide the egg salad mixture evenly among the toast slices, spreading it out to cover the surface.
5. If desired, top each open-faced sandwich with sliced tomatoes, avocado, lettuce, or sprouts for extra flavor and nutrition.
6. Serve immediately and enjoy!

Chicken Caesar Salad with Light Dressing

Ingredients:

For the Salad:

- 2 boneless, skinless chicken breasts
- Salt and pepper to taste
- 1 tablespoon olive oil
- 1 head romaine lettuce, chopped
- 1/4 cup grated Parmesan cheese
- Whole wheat croutons (optional)
- Cherry tomatoes, halved (optional)

For the Light Dressing:

- 1/4 cup plain Greek yogurt
- 2 tablespoons grated Parmesan cheese

- 1 tablespoon lemon juice
- 1 teaspoon Dijon mustard
- 1 clove garlic, minced
- Salt and pepper to taste
- Water (to thin, if needed)

Directions:

1. Preheat the grill or a grill pan over medium-high heat.
2. Season the chicken breasts with salt and pepper.
3. Drizzle olive oil over the chicken breasts, rubbing to coat evenly.
4. Grill the chicken breasts for 6-8 minutes per side, or until cooked through and no longer pink in the center. Remove from heat and let them rest for a few minutes before slicing.
5. In a large mixing bowl, combine the chopped romaine lettuce and grated Parmesan cheese.
6. To make the light dressing, in a small bowl, whisk together the Greek yogurt, grated Parmesan cheese, lemon juice, Dijon mustard, minced garlic, salt, and pepper. If the dressing is too thick, add a splash of water to thin it to your desired consistency.
7. Add the sliced grilled chicken breasts to the bowl with the romaine lettuce.
8. Drizzle the light dressing over the salad and toss to coat evenly.
9. Divide the salad among serving plates.
10. Optionally, top each salad with whole wheat croutons and cherry tomatoes.
11. Serve immediately and enjoy!

Chickpea Salad Sandwich on Whole-Wheat Bread

Ingredients:

- 1 can (15 oz) chickpeas (garbanzo beans), drained and rinsed
- 1/4 cup diced red onion
- 1/4 cup diced celery
- 1/4 cup diced bell pepper (any color)
- 2 tablespoons chopped fresh parsley or cilantro
- 2 tablespoons plain Greek yogurt or mayonnaise (choose low-fat or light options if desired)
- 1 tablespoon lemon juice
- 1 teaspoon Dijon mustard
- Salt and pepper to taste
- 4 slices whole wheat bread, toasted
- Lettuce leaves, tomato slices, and avocado slices for topping (optional)

Directions:

1. In a large mixing bowl, mash the chickpeas with a fork or potato masher until they are slightly chunky.
2. Add diced red onion, diced celery, diced bell pepper, chopped fresh parsley or cilantro, Greek yogurt or mayonnaise, lemon juice, Dijon mustard, salt, and pepper to the bowl.
3. Mix all the ingredients until well combined.
4. Taste and adjust seasoning as needed.
5. Divide the chickpea salad mixture evenly among the toasted whole wheat bread slices.
6. Top each sandwich with lettuce leaves, tomato slices, and avocado slices if desired.
7. Serve immediately and enjoy!

Black Bean Burgers with Sweet Potato Fries

Black Bean Burgers

Ingredients:

- 1 can (15 oz) black beans, drained and rinsed
- 1/2 cup cooked quinoa or breadcrumbs
- 1/4 cup diced red onion
- 1/4 cup diced bell pepper (any color)
- 2 cloves garlic, minced
- 1 teaspoon ground cumin
- 1 teaspoon chili powder
- 1/2 teaspoon smoked paprika
- Salt and pepper to taste
- 1 egg, beaten (or flaxseed meal mixed with water for a vegan option)
- 1 tablespoon olive oil

For Serving:

- Whole wheat burger buns
- Lettuce leaves
- Tomato slices
- Avocado slices
- Mustard, ketchup, or your favorite burger toppings

Sweet Potato Fries

Ingredients:

- 2 medium sweet potatoes, peeled and cut into fries
- 1 tablespoon olive oil
- 1 teaspoon garlic powder
- 1 teaspoon smoked paprika
- Salt and pepper to taste

Directions:

1. Preheat the oven to 400°F (200°C).
2. In a large mixing bowl, mash the black beans with a fork or potato masher until mostly smooth, leaving some chunks for texture.
3. Add cooked quinoa or breadcrumbs, diced red onion, diced bell pepper, minced garlic, ground cumin, chili powder, smoked paprika, salt, and pepper to the bowl. Mix until well combined.
4. Add the beaten egg to the mixture and stir until everything is evenly incorporated. If the mixture is too wet, you can add more quinoa or breadcrumbs to bind it together.
5. Divide the mixture into 4 equal portions and shape each portion into a burger patty.
6. Heat olive oil in a skillet over medium heat. Cook the black bean burgers for 4-5 minutes on each side, or until golden brown and heated through.
7. While the burgers are cooking, prepare the sweet potato fries. In a large mixing bowl, toss the sweet potato fries with olive oil, garlic powder, smoked paprika, salt, and pepper until evenly coated.
8. Spread the sweet potato fries in a single layer on a baking sheet lined with parchment paper.
9. Bake the sweet potato fries in the preheated oven for 20-25 minutes, flipping halfway through, until golden and crispy.
10. Assemble the black bean burgers by placing each burger patty on a whole wheat bun and topping with lettuce, tomato slices, avocado slices, and your favorite burger toppings.
11. Serve the black bean burgers with the crispy sweet potato fries on the side and enjoy!

Tuna Poke Bowl with Brown Rice and Edamame

Ingredients:

For the Tuna Poke:

- 2 (6 oz) sushi-grade tuna steaks, diced into bite-sized pieces
- 2 tablespoons soy sauce (reduced-sodium if preferred)
- 1 tablespoon sesame oil
- 1 tablespoon rice vinegar
- 1 teaspoon grated fresh ginger
- 1 teaspoon honey or maple syrup
- 1 green onion, thinly sliced
- 1 tablespoon sesame seeds
- Optional toppings: sliced avocado, cucumber, radishes, seaweed salad

For the Bowl:

- 2 cups cooked brown rice
- 1 cup shelled edamame, cooked according to package instructions
- 1/2 cup shredded carrots
- 1/2 cup thinly sliced red cabbage
- 1/4 cup sliced green onions
- 1/4 cup sliced radishes
- Optional garnish: pickled ginger, wasabi, nori strips

Directions:

1. In a medium bowl, whisk together soy sauce, sesame oil, rice vinegar, grated ginger, and honey or maple syrup to make the marinade for the tuna poke.

2. Add diced tuna to the marinade and gently toss until evenly coated. Cover and refrigerate for at least 15-30 minutes to allow the flavors to meld.

3. While the tuna is marinating, prepare the brown rice according to package instructions, and cook the shelled edamame.

4. Once the tuna is marinated, assemble the poke bowl by dividing cooked brown rice among serving bowls.

5. Top the brown rice with marinated tuna poke.

6. Arrange shelled edamame, shredded carrots, thinly sliced red cabbage, sliced green onions, and sliced radishes around the tuna poke.

7. Garnish the bowl with sliced avocado, cucumber, radishes, seaweed salad, pickled ginger, wasabi, and nori strips if desired.

8. Sprinkle sesame seeds over the poke bowl for added crunch and flavor.

9. Serve immediately and enjoy your Tuna Poke Bowl with Brown Rice and Edamame!

Turkey Chili with a Dollop of Greek Yogurt

Ingredients:

- 1 tablespoon olive oil
- 1 onion, chopped
- 2 cloves garlic, minced
- 1 bell pepper, diced
- 1 pound ground turkey
- 1 can (15 oz) diced tomatoes
- 1 can (15 oz) kidney beans, drained and rinsed
- 1 can (15 oz) black beans, drained and rinsed
- 1 cup corn kernels (fresh, frozen, or canned)
- 1 cup low-sodium chicken broth or vegetable broth
- 2 tablespoons chili powder
- 1 teaspoon ground cumin

- 1/2 teaspoon smoked paprika
- Salt and pepper to taste
- Greek yogurt for serving
- Optional toppings: chopped fresh cilantro, sliced green onions, shredded cheese, avocado slices

Directions:

1. Heat olive oil in a large pot over medium heat. Add chopped onion, minced garlic, and diced bell pepper. Cook, stirring occasionally, until vegetables are softened, about 5 minutes.
2. Add ground turkey to the pot. Cook, breaking up the meat with a spoon, until browned and cooked through, about 5-7 minutes.
3. Stir in diced tomatoes, kidney beans, black beans, corn kernels, chicken broth, chili powder, ground cumin, smoked paprika, salt, and pepper.
4. Bring the chili to a simmer, then reduce heat to low. Cover and let it simmer for about 20-25 minutes, stirring occasionally, to allow the flavors to meld and the chili to thicken.
5. Taste and adjust seasoning as needed.
6. Ladle the turkey chili into serving bowls. Top each bowl with a dollop of Greek yogurt.
7. Garnish with chopped fresh cilantro, sliced green onions, shredded cheese, and avocado slices if desired.
8. Serve hot and enjoy your hearty Turkey Chili with a dollop of Greek Yogurt!

Shrimp Scampi with Zucchini Noodles

Ingredients:

- 1 lb large shrimp, peeled and deveined

- 4 medium zucchinis, spiralized into noodles
- 3 tablespoons olive oil
- 4 cloves garlic, minced
- 1/4 teaspoon red pepper flakes (optional)
- 1/4 cup dry white wine (or chicken broth)
- Juice of 1 lemon
- Salt and pepper to taste
- 2 tablespoons chopped fresh parsley
- Grated Parmesan cheese for serving (optional)

Directions:

1. Heat 2 tablespoons of olive oil in a large skillet over medium heat. Add the minced garlic and red pepper flakes (if using), and cook for about 1 minute, until fragrant.
2. Add the shrimp to the skillet and cook for 2-3 minutes per side, until pink and opaque. Remove the shrimp from the skillet and set aside.
3. In the same skillet, add the remaining tablespoon of olive oil. Add the spiralized zucchini noodles and cook for 2-3 minutes, tossing occasionally, until just tender.
4. Return the cooked shrimp to the skillet with the zucchini noodles.
5. Pour in the white wine (or chicken broth) and lemon juice. Cook for 1-2 minutes, until heated through and slightly reduced.
6. Season the shrimp scampi with salt and pepper to taste.
7. Remove the skillet from heat and sprinkle chopped fresh parsley over the shrimp scampi.
8. Serve the shrimp scampi over zucchini noodles immediately, garnished with grated Parmesan cheese if desired.
9. Enjoy your light and flavorful Shrimp Scampi with Zucchini Noodles!

Chicken and Vegetable Skewers with Peanut Sauce

Ingredients:

For the Skewers:

- 1 lb boneless, skinless chicken breasts, cut into cubes
- 1 red bell pepper, cut into chunks
- 1 yellow bell pepper, cut into chunks
- 1 zucchini, sliced into rounds
- 1 red onion, cut into chunks
- Wooden skewers, soaked in water for 30 minutes

For the Marinade:

- 2 tablespoons soy sauce (reduced-sodium if preferred)
- 2 tablespoons olive oil
- 2 cloves garlic, minced
- 1 teaspoon grated ginger
- 1 tablespoon honey or maple syrup
- Salt and pepper to taste

For the Peanut Sauce:

- 1/4 cup creamy peanut butter
- 2 tablespoons soy sauce (reduced-sodium if preferred)
- 1 tablespoon rice vinegar
- 1 tablespoon honey or maple syrup
- 1 clove garlic, minced
- 1 teaspoon grated ginger
- 2-4 tablespoons water, to thin as needed

Directions:

1. In a small bowl, whisk together the ingredients for the marinade: soy sauce, olive oil, minced garlic, grated ginger, honey or maple syrup, salt, and pepper.

2. Place the cubed chicken breasts in a shallow dish or resealable plastic bag. Pour the marinade over the chicken and toss to coat. Cover and refrigerate for at least 30 minutes, or up to 4 hours.

3. Preheat the grill or grill pan over medium-high heat.

4. Thread the marinated chicken cubes, bell pepper chunks, zucchini rounds, and red onion chunks onto the soaked wooden skewers, alternating between the ingredients.

5. Grill the skewers for 8-10 minutes, turning occasionally, until the chicken is cooked through and the vegetables are tender and lightly charred.

6. While the skewers are grilling, prepare the peanut sauce. In a small saucepan, combine peanut butter, soy sauce, rice vinegar, honey or maple syrup, minced garlic, and grated ginger. Heat over low heat, stirring constantly, until the peanut butter is melted and the sauce is smooth. Add water as needed to thin the sauce to your desired consistency.

7. Serve the grilled chicken and vegetable skewers hot, with the peanut sauce on the side for dipping or drizzling.

8. Enjoy your delicious Chicken and Vegetable Skewers with Peanut Sauce!

Lentil and Veggie Stuffed Peppers

Ingredients:

- 4 large bell peppers, any color
- 1 cup dry brown or green lentils, rinsed
- 2 cups vegetable broth or water
- 1 tablespoon olive oil
- 1 onion, diced
- 2 cloves garlic, minced
- 1 carrot, diced
- 1 zucchini, diced
- 1 cup diced tomatoes (fresh or canned)
- 1 teaspoon dried oregano
- 1 teaspoon dried basil
- Salt and pepper to taste
- 1/2 cup shredded mozzarella or Parmesan cheese (optional)
- Fresh parsley or basil for garnish (optional)

Directions:

1. Preheat the oven to 375°F (190°C). Grease a baking dish large enough to fit the bell peppers.
2. Cut the tops off the bell peppers and remove the seeds and membranes. Place the hollowed-out bell peppers in the prepared baking dish, cut side up.
3. In a medium saucepan, combine the rinsed lentils and vegetable broth or water. Bring to a boil, then reduce heat to low, cover, and simmer for 20-25 minutes, or until the lentils are tender and the liquid is absorbed.
4. In a large skillet, heat olive oil over medium heat. Add diced onion and minced garlic, and cook until softened and fragrant, about 2-3 minutes.

5. Add diced carrot and zucchini to the skillet, and cook for another 5 minutes, or until the vegetables are tender.

6. Stir in diced tomatoes, dried oregano, dried basil, cooked lentils, salt, and pepper. Cook for an additional 2-3 minutes, until heated through and well combined.

7. If using, stir in shredded mozzarella or Parmesan cheese until melted and incorporated into the lentil and veggie mixture.

8. Spoon the lentil and veggie mixture into the hollowed-out bell peppers, pressing down gently to pack the filling.

9. Cover the baking dish with aluminum foil and bake in the preheated oven for 25-30 minutes, or until the bell peppers are tender.

10. Remove the foil and bake for an additional 5-10 minutes, or until the tops are slightly golden and the cheese is bubbly (if using).

11. Garnish with fresh parsley or basil, if desired, and serve hot.

12. Enjoy your delicious Lentil and Veggie Stuffed Peppers!

Cobb Salad with Grilled Chicken and Light Vinaigrette

Ingredients:

For the Salad:

- 2 boneless, skinless chicken breasts
- Salt and pepper to taste
- 1 tablespoon olive oil
- 6 cups mixed salad greens (such as romaine lettuce or spinach)
- 4 hard-boiled eggs, sliced
- 1 cup cherry tomatoes, halved
- 1 avocado, diced

- 4 slices cooked bacon, crumbled
- 1/2 cup crumbled blue cheese (optional)

For the Light Vinaigrette:

- 3 tablespoons extra virgin olive oil
- 2 tablespoons red wine vinegar
- 1 teaspoon Dijon mustard
- 1 clove garlic, minced
- 1/2 teaspoon dried oregano
- Salt and pepper to taste

Directions:

1. Preheat a grill or grill pan over medium-high heat.
2. Season the chicken breasts with salt and pepper on both sides.
3. Drizzle olive oil over the chicken breasts, rubbing to coat evenly.
4. Grill the chicken breasts for 6-8 minutes per side, or until cooked through and no longer pink in the center. Remove from heat and let them rest for a few minutes before slicing.
5. While the chicken is grilling, prepare the salad ingredients: wash and dry the mixed salad greens, slice the hard-boiled eggs, halve the cherry tomatoes, dice the avocado, and crumble the cooked bacon.
6. In a small bowl, whisk together the ingredients for the light vinaigrette: extra virgin olive oil, red wine vinegar, Dijon mustard, minced garlic, dried oregano, salt, and pepper.
7. To assemble the Cobb Salad, divide the mixed salad greens among serving plates.
8. Arrange sliced grilled chicken, hard-boiled egg slices, halved cherry tomatoes, diced avocado, crumbled bacon, and crumbled blue cheese (if using) over the salad greens.
9. Drizzle the light vinaigrette over the salad just before serving.
10. Serve immediately and enjoy your delicious Cobb Salad with Grilled Chicken and Light Vinaigrette!

Chapter 6: Snack and Dessert Recipes

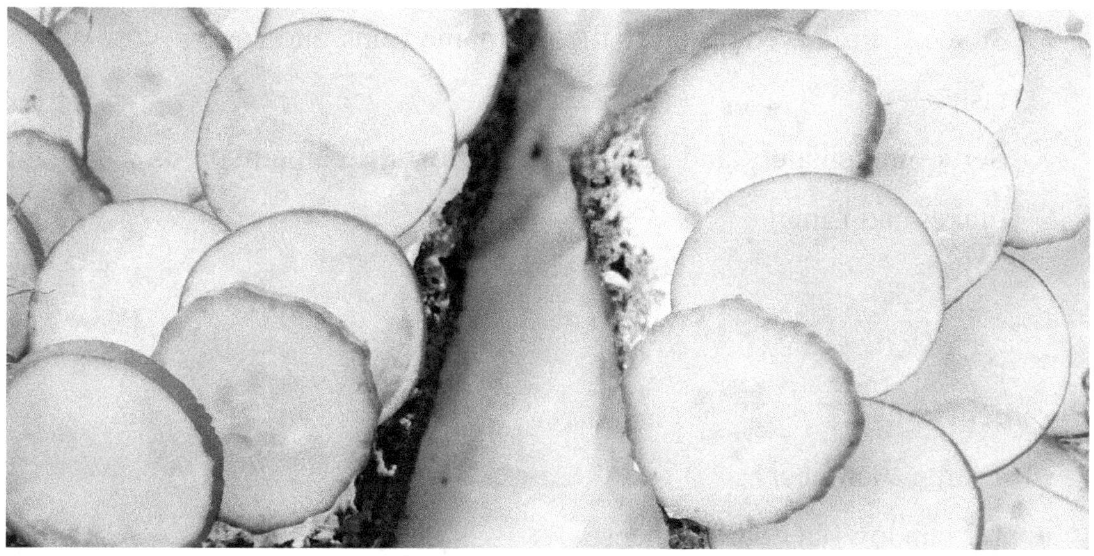

Edamame Pods with Chili Flakes and Lime

Ingredients:

- 2 cups edamame pods (fresh or frozen)
- 1 tablespoon olive oil
- 1/2 teaspoon chili flakes (adjust to taste)
- 1 lime, cut into wedges
- Salt to taste

Directions:

1. If using frozen edamame pods, thaw them according to package instructions. If using fresh edamame pods, rinse them under cold water.
2. Heat olive oil in a large skillet over medium heat.
3. Add the edamame pods to the skillet and sauté for 5-7 minutes, stirring occasionally, until heated through.
4. Sprinkle chili flakes over the edamame pods and continue to cook for another 2-3 minutes, stirring frequently, until fragrant.

5. Remove the skillet from heat and transfer the edamame pods to a serving plate.

6. Squeeze lime wedges over the edamame pods and season with salt to taste.

7. Serve immediately and enjoy your flavorful Edamame Pods with Chili Flakes and Lime!

Cucumber Slices with Cottage Cheese and Dill

Ingredients:

- 1 large cucumber
- 1/2 cup low-fat cottage cheese
- 1 tablespoon fresh dill, chopped
- Salt and pepper to taste

Directions:

1. Wash the cucumber thoroughly under cold water and pat it dry with a paper towel.

2. Slice the cucumber into thin rounds using a sharp knife or a mandoline slicer.

3. In a small bowl, combine the low-fat cottage cheese and chopped fresh dill. Mix well.

4. Arrange the cucumber slices on a serving platter or individual plates.

5. Spoon a dollop of the cottage cheese mixture onto each cucumber slice.

6. Sprinkle salt and pepper over the cucumber slices with cottage cheese.

7. Garnish with additional fresh dill, if desired.

8. Serve immediately and enjoy your light and refreshing Cucumber Slices with Cottage Cheese and Dill!

Roasted Chickpeas with Rosemary and Garlic

Ingredients:

- 1 can (15 oz) chickpeas (garbanzo beans), drained and rinsed
- 1 tablespoon olive oil
- 2 cloves garlic, minced
- 1 tablespoon fresh rosemary, chopped (or 1 teaspoon dried rosemary)
- Salt and pepper to taste

Directions:

1. Preheat your oven to 400°F (200°C) and line a baking sheet with parchment paper.
2. Pat the rinsed chickpeas dry with a paper towel and spread them out on the prepared baking sheet.
3. Drizzle olive oil over the chickpeas and toss to coat evenly.
4. Sprinkle minced garlic and chopped rosemary over the chickpeas, and toss again to distribute the seasonings.
5. Spread the seasoned chickpeas out in a single layer on the baking sheet.
6. Roast in the preheated oven for 20-25 minutes, stirring halfway through, until the chickpeas are golden brown and crispy.
7. Remove the baking sheet from the oven and let the roasted chickpeas cool slightly.
8. Season with salt and pepper to taste.
9. Serve the roasted chickpeas with rosemary and garlic as a crunchy and flavorful snack.

Apple Slices with Almond Butter and Cinnamon

Ingredients:

- 1 medium apple (such as Granny Smith or Honeycrisp)
- 2 tablespoons almond butter (unsweetened)
- 1/2 teaspoon ground cinnamon

Directions:

1. Wash the apple thoroughly under cold water and pat it dry with a paper towel.
2. Core the apple and slice it into thin wedges using a sharp knife.
3. Arrange the apple slices on a serving plate or individual plates.
4. In a small microwave-safe bowl, heat the almond butter in the microwave for 20-30 seconds, or until slightly softened.
5. Drizzle the warm almond butter over the apple slices.
6. Sprinkle ground cinnamon over the almond butter-topped apple slices.
7. Serve immediately and enjoy your delicious Apple Slices with Almond Butter and Cinnamon!

Bell Pepper Strips with Guacamole

Ingredients:

- 2 bell peppers (any color), sliced into strips
- 2 ripe avocados
- 1 small tomato, diced
- 1/4 cup red onion, finely chopped
- 1 clove garlic, minced
- 1 tablespoon fresh lime juice
- Salt and pepper to taste

- Optional toppings: chopped cilantro, sliced jalapeño, diced red onion

Directions:

1. Wash the bell peppers thoroughly under cold water and pat them dry with a paper towel. Remove the stems and seeds, then slice them into thin strips.
2. In a medium bowl, scoop out the flesh of the avocados and mash them with a fork until smooth.
3. Add diced tomato, chopped red onion, minced garlic, and fresh lime juice to the mashed avocados. Mix well to combine.
4. Season the guacamole with salt and pepper to taste. Adjust seasoning as needed.
5. Arrange the bell pepper strips on a serving platter.
6. Serve the bell pepper strips with the guacamole for dipping.
7. Garnish with optional toppings such as chopped cilantro, sliced jalapeño, or diced red onion if desired.
8. Enjoy your flavorful Bell Pepper Strips with Guacamole!

Greek Yogurt with Berries and Chia Seeds

Ingredients:

- 1/2 cup Greek yogurt (low-fat or non-fat)
- 1/4 cup mixed berries (such as strawberries, blueberries, raspberries)
- 1 tablespoon chia seeds

Directions:

1. In a small bowl or serving glass, spoon Greek yogurt.
2. Top with mixed berries and chia seeds.
3. Serve immediately and enjoy your protein-rich and fiber-filled Greek Yogurt with Berries and Chia Seeds!

Turkey Roll-Ups with Mustard and Lettuce Wraps

Ingredients:

- 4 slices of turkey breast (nitrate-free)
- 2 tablespoons mustard (choose low-sodium)
- 4 large lettuce leaves (such as romaine or iceberg)
- Optional: sliced cucumber, tomato, avocado

Directions:

1. Lay out the turkey slices on a clean surface.
2. Spread mustard evenly over each turkey slice.
3. Place a lettuce leaf on top of each turkey slice.
4. Add any optional ingredients such as sliced cucumber, tomato, or avocado on top of the lettuce leaf.
5. Roll up the turkey slices tightly, enclosing the lettuce and any additional fillings.
6. Secure the rolls with toothpicks if necessary.
7. Serve immediately and enjoy your Turkey Roll-Ups with Mustard and Lettuce Wraps!

Sliced Pear with a dollop of Ricotta Cheese and a drizzle of Honey

Ingredients:

- 1 ripe pear, thinly sliced
- 2 tablespoons part-skim ricotta cheese
- 1 teaspoon raw honey

Directions:

1. Wash the pear thoroughly under cold water and pat it dry with a paper towel. Remove the core and slice it thinly.
2. Arrange the pear slices on a serving plate or individual plates.
3. Place a dollop of part-skim ricotta cheese on each pear slice.
4. Drizzle raw honey over the ricotta cheese and pear slices.
5. Serve immediately and enjoy your healthy Sliced Pear with Ricotta Cheese and Honey!

Carrot Sticks with Hummus

Ingredients:

- 2 medium carrots, peeled and cut into sticks
- 1/4 cup hummus (choose low-fat or homemade)

Directions:

1. Wash the carrots thoroughly under cold water and peel them.
2. Cut the carrots into sticks.
3. Arrange the carrot sticks on a serving plate.
4. Serve with hummus for dipping.
5. Enjoy your healthy Carrot Sticks with Hummus!

Roasted Pumpkin Seeds

Ingredients:

- 1 cup raw pumpkin seeds (also known as pepitas)
- 1 tablespoon olive oil
- 1/2 teaspoon sea salt (or to taste)
- Optional seasonings: garlic powder, onion powder, paprika, cayenne pepper

Directions:

1. Preheat your oven to 300°F (150°C) and line a baking sheet with parchment paper.
2. Rinse the pumpkin seeds under cold water to remove any pulp or strings. Pat them dry with a paper towel.
3. In a bowl, toss the pumpkin seeds with olive oil until evenly coated.
4. Spread the pumpkin seeds out in a single layer on the prepared baking sheet.
5. Sprinkle sea salt over the pumpkin seeds, along with any optional seasonings you desire.
6. Roast the pumpkin seeds in the preheated oven for 20-25 minutes, stirring occasionally, until they are golden brown and crispy.
7. Remove the baking sheet from the oven and let the pumpkin seeds cool completely before serving.
8. Enjoy your healthy Roasted Pumpkin Seeds as a crunchy and nutritious snack!

Seaweed Snacks

Ingredients:

- 4 sheets of roasted seaweed (nori)
- 1 tablespoon sesame oil
- 1 teaspoon soy sauce (low-sodium if preferred)
- Optional: sesame seeds, chili flakes, wasabi powder

Directions:

1. Lay the seaweed sheets flat on a cutting board.
2. In a small bowl, mix together sesame oil and soy sauce.

3. Using a pastry brush, lightly brush the mixture onto one side of each seaweed sheet.

4. Sprinkle sesame seeds, chili flakes, or wasabi powder over the seaweed sheets if desired.

5. Carefully cut each seaweed sheet into smaller squares or rectangles using a sharp knife or kitchen scissors.

6. Serve immediately and enjoy your homemade Seaweed Snacks!

Air-Popped Popcorn with Nutritional Yeast

Ingredients:

- 1/4 cup popcorn kernels
- 1-2 tablespoons nutritional yeast
- Optional: salt, pepper, garlic powder, onion powder, paprika (to taste)

Directions:

1. Using an air popper, pop the popcorn kernels according to the manufacturer's instructions until all the kernels are popped.

2. Transfer the popped popcorn to a large bowl.

3. Sprinkle nutritional yeast evenly over the popcorn while it's still warm.

4. Add optional seasonings such as salt, pepper, garlic powder, onion powder, or paprika according to your taste preferences.

5. Toss the popcorn gently to evenly distribute the nutritional yeast and seasonings.

6. Serve immediately and enjoy your Air-Popped Popcorn with Nutritional Yeast!

Sliced Bell Peppers with cottage cheese

Ingredients:

- 2 bell peppers (any color), sliced into strips
- 1/2 cup low-fat cottage cheese
- Optional: salt, pepper, herbs (to taste)

Directions:

1. Wash the bell peppers thoroughly under cold water and pat them dry with a paper towel. Remove the stems and seeds, then slice them into strips.
2. Arrange the bell pepper strips on a serving plate or individual plates.
3. Spoon low-fat cottage cheese into a small bowl.
4. Optional: season the cottage cheese with a pinch of salt, pepper, or your favorite herbs, such as basil or dill.
5. Serve the bell pepper strips with the seasoned cottage cheese for dipping.
6. Enjoy your Sliced Bell Peppers with Cottage Cheese as a healthy and satisfying snack!

Sugar-Snap Peas with a dollop of Peanut Butter

Ingredients:

- 1 cup sugar snap peas
- 2 tablespoons peanut butter (unsweetened)

Directions:

1. Wash the sugar snap peas thoroughly under cold water and pat them dry with a paper towel.
2. Arrange the sugar snap peas on a serving plate.

3. Spoon peanut butter into a small bowl.

4. Optional: warm the peanut butter in the microwave for a few seconds to make it easier to drizzle.

5. Drizzle the peanut butter over the sugar snap peas or place a dollop of peanut butter on the side for dipping.

6. Enjoy your Sugar Snap Peas with Peanut Butter as a healthy and satisfying snack!

Spiced Baked Pears with Berries

Ingredients:

- 2 ripe but firm pears, halved and cored
- 1/4 teaspoon ground cinnamon
- 1/8 teaspoon ground nutmeg
- 1/8 teaspoon ground ginger
- 1 tablespoon honey (optional)
- 1/4 cup mixed berries (such as blueberries, raspberries, blackberries)

Directions:

1. Preheat your oven to 375°F (190°C) and line a baking dish with parchment paper.

2. In a small bowl, mix together the ground cinnamon, nutmeg, and ginger.

3. Place the pear halves, cut side up, in the prepared baking dish.

4. Sprinkle the spice mixture evenly over the pear halves.

5. Drizzle honey over the pear halves, if using.

6. Bake in the preheated oven for 20-25 minutes, or until the pears are tender and lightly caramelized.

7. Remove the pears from the oven and let them cool slightly.

8. Once cooled, top each pear half with mixed berries.

9. Serve warm and enjoy your Spiced Baked Pears with Berries!

Dark Chocolate Avocado Mousse

Ingredients:

- 2 ripe avocados
- 1/4 cup unsweetened cocoa powder
- 1/4 cup maple syrup or honey (adjust to taste)
- 1 teaspoon vanilla extract
- Pinch of salt
- 1/4 cup almond milk or coconut milk (unsweetened)
- Optional toppings: fresh berries, chopped nuts, shredded coconut

Directions:

1. Cut the avocados in half, remove the pits, and scoop the flesh into a blender or food processor.
2. Add cocoa powder, maple syrup or honey, vanilla extract, salt, and almond milk to the blender.
3. Blend until smooth and creamy, scraping down the sides of the blender as needed to ensure everything is well combined.
4. Taste the mousse and adjust sweetness if needed by adding more maple syrup or honey.
5. Transfer the mousse into serving bowls or glasses.
6. Cover and refrigerate for at least 30 minutes to allow the mousse to chill and set.
7. Before serving, top with fresh berries, chopped nuts, or shredded coconut if desired.
8. Serve and enjoy your delicious Dark Chocolate Avocado Mousse!

Frozen Yogurt Bark with Berries and Nuts

Ingredients:

- 1 cup Greek yogurt (low-fat or non-fat)
- 1 tablespoon honey or maple syrup (optional, adjust to taste)
- 1/2 teaspoon vanilla extract
- 1/4 cup mixed berries (such as strawberries, blueberries, raspberries)
- 2 tablespoons chopped nuts (such as almonds, walnuts)

Directions:

1. In a mixing bowl, combine Greek yogurt, honey or maple syrup (if using), and vanilla extract. Stir until well combined.
2. Line a baking sheet with parchment paper or wax paper.
3. Pour the Greek yogurt mixture onto the lined baking sheet, spreading it out evenly into a thin layer.
4. Sprinkle mixed berries and chopped nuts over the Greek yogurt layer, pressing them gently into the yogurt.
5. Place the baking sheet in the freezer and freeze for at least 2-3 hours, or until the yogurt bark is completely frozen.
6. Once frozen, remove the baking sheet from the freezer and break the yogurt bark into pieces using your hands or a knife.
7. Serve immediately and enjoy your Frozen Yogurt Bark with Berries and Nuts!

No-Bake Cheesecake Bars with Almond Crust (Sweetened with Dates)

Ingredients:

For the Almond Crust:

- 1 cup almonds
- 1 cup pitted dates
- Pinch of salt

For the Cheesecake Filling:

- 2 cups Greek yogurt (low-fat or non-fat)
- 8 ounces cream cheese (softened)
- 1/4 cup honey or maple syrup (adjust to taste)
- 1 teaspoon vanilla extract
- Zest of 1 lemon (optional)
- Fresh berries for topping (optional)

Directions:

1. In a food processor, combine almonds, pitted dates, and a pinch of salt. Pulse until the mixture forms a sticky dough.
2. Line a square baking dish with parchment paper. Press the almond mixture evenly into the bottom of the dish to form the crust. Place in the refrigerator while you prepare the filling.
3. In a mixing bowl, beat together Greek yogurt, softened cream cheese, honey or maple syrup, vanilla extract, and lemon zest (if using) until smooth and creamy.
4. Pour the cheesecake filling over the almond crust in the baking dish, spreading it out evenly.

5. Cover the baking dish with plastic wrap and refrigerate for at least 4 hours, or until the cheesecake filling is set.

6. Once set, remove the cheesecake from the refrigerator and slice into bars.

7. Serve the no-bake cheesecake bars topped with fresh berries if desired.

8. Enjoy your delicious No-Bake Cheesecake Bars with Almond Crust sweetened with dates!

Fruit and Nut Snack Mix with a touch of dark chocolate

Ingredients:

- 1 cup mixed nuts (such as almonds, walnuts, cashews)
- 1/2 cup dried fruit (such as cranberries, raisins, apricots)
- 1/4 cup dark chocolate chips or chunks (at least 70% cocoa)
- Optional: 1/4 teaspoon sea salt

Directions:

1. In a large bowl, combine mixed nuts and dried fruit.

2. Add dark chocolate chips or chunks to the bowl.

3. If desired, sprinkle sea salt over the mixture for a sweet and salty contrast.

4. Toss everything together until the nuts, fruit, and chocolate are evenly distributed.

5. Transfer the snack mix to an airtight container or portion it into individual snack bags for easy grab-and-go access.

6. Enjoy your delicious Fruit and Nut Snack Mix with Dark Chocolate as a healthy and satisfying snack!

Mini Crustless Pumpkin Pies

Ingredients:

- 1 cup canned pumpkin puree (not pumpkin pie filling)
- 1/2 cup low-fat milk or unsweetened almond milk
- 2 large eggs
- 1/4 cup honey or maple syrup
- 1 teaspoon vanilla extract
- 1 teaspoon ground cinnamon
- 1/2 teaspoon ground ginger
- 1/4 teaspoon ground nutmeg
- 1/4 teaspoon ground cloves
- Optional: Whipped cream or Greek yogurt for serving

Directions:

1. Preheat your oven to 350°F (175°C) and grease a muffin tin with cooking spray or line it with paper liners.
2. In a large mixing bowl, whisk together the pumpkin puree, milk, eggs, honey or maple syrup, and vanilla extract until smooth.
3. Add the ground cinnamon, ground ginger, ground nutmeg, and ground cloves to the bowl, and whisk until well combined.
4. Pour the pumpkin mixture evenly into the prepared muffin tin, filling each cup almost to the top.
5. Bake in the preheated oven for 20-25 minutes, or until the pies are set and a toothpick inserted into the center comes out clean.
6. Remove the mini pumpkin pies from the oven and let them cool in the muffin tin for 10 minutes.
7. After cooling, carefully remove the mini pies from the muffin tin and transfer them to a wire rack to cool completely.

8. Once cooled, serve the mini crustless pumpkin pies topped with whipped cream or Greek yogurt if desired.

9. Enjoy your delicious Mini Crustless Pumpkin Pies as a healthier alternative to traditional pumpkin pie!

Strawberry-Chia Seed Jam on Whole-Wheat Toast

Ingredients:

- 2 cups fresh strawberries, hulled and chopped
- 2 tablespoons chia seeds
- 1-2 tablespoons honey or maple syrup (optional, adjust to taste)
- 1 teaspoon vanilla extract

Directions:

1. In a small saucepan, combine chopped strawberries, chia seeds, honey or maple syrup (if using), and vanilla extract.

2. Cook over medium heat, stirring occasionally, until the strawberries begin to break down and the mixture thickens, about 5-7 minutes.

3. Use a fork or potato masher to mash the strawberries to your desired consistency.

4. Continue to cook for another 2-3 minutes, or until the jam reaches your desired thickness.

5. Remove the saucepan from the heat and let the jam cool to room temperature.

6. Once cooled, transfer the jam to a clean jar or container and refrigerate for at least 1 hour to allow it to set.

7. Spread the strawberry-chia seed jam generously on whole-wheat toast or your favorite bread.

8. Enjoy your delicious Strawberry-Chia Seed Jam on Whole-Wheat Toast as a nutritious and satisfying breakfast or snack!

Microwave Mug Brownie

Ingredients:

- 2 tablespoons all-purpose flour
- 2 tablespoons unsweetened cocoa powder
- 2 tablespoons granulated sugar
- Pinch of salt
- 2 tablespoons milk (dairy or plant-based)
- 1 tablespoon vegetable oil or melted butter
- 1/4 teaspoon vanilla extract
- Optional add-ins: chocolate chips, chopped nuts, or a dollop of nut butter

Directions:

1. In a microwave-safe mug, whisk together the all-purpose flour, unsweetened cocoa powder, granulated sugar, and salt until well combined.
2. Add the milk, vegetable oil or melted butter, and vanilla extract to the mug. Stir until the mixture is smooth and no lumps remain.
3. If desired, fold in chocolate chips, chopped nuts, or a dollop of nut butter for added flavor and texture.
4. Microwave the mug brownie on high for 60-90 seconds, or until the brownie is set and cooked through. Cooking time may vary depending on the wattage of your microwave, so adjust as needed.
5. Carefully remove the mug from the microwave (it will be hot) and let the brownie cool for a minute or two before enjoying.
6. Optionally, top the brownie with a scoop of vanilla ice cream or a drizzle of chocolate sauce for extra indulgence.

Chapter 7: Dinner Recipes

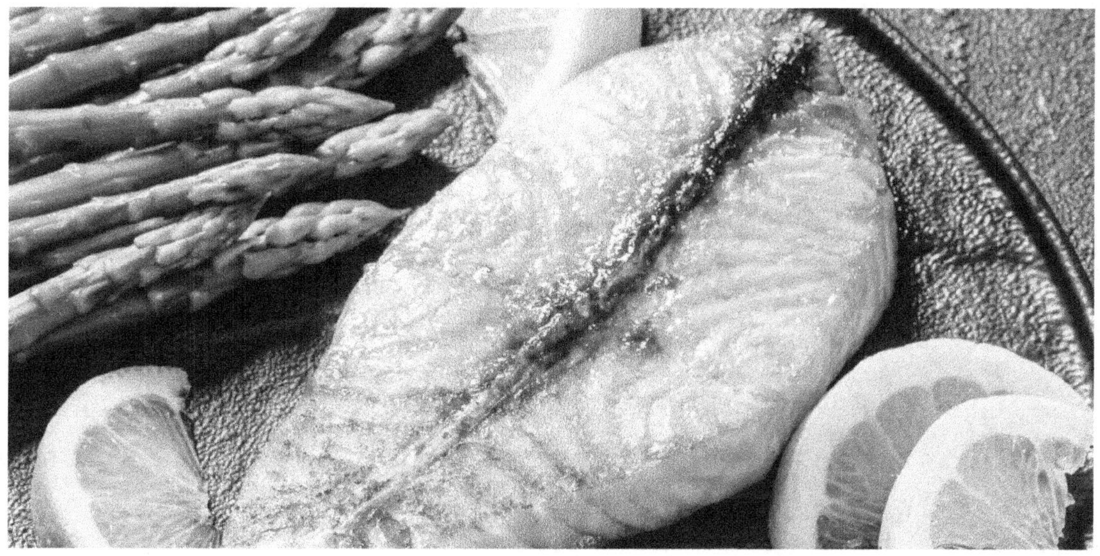

Salmon with Lemon Dill Sauce and Roasted Asparagus

Salmon with Lemon Dill Sauce:

Ingredients:

- 4 salmon filets (about 4-6 ounces each), skin removed
- 2 tablespoons olive oil
- Salt and pepper to taste
- 2 tablespoons chopped fresh dill
- 1 lemon, juiced
- 2 cloves garlic, minced
- 1/4 cup plain Greek yogurt (low-fat or non-fat)
- Lemon wedges for serving

Roasted Asparagus:

Ingredients:

- 1 bunch asparagus, tough ends trimmed
- 1 tablespoon olive oil
- Salt and pepper to taste
- Lemon zest (optional)

Directions:

1. Preheat the oven to 400°F (200°C).
2. Prepare the salmon:
    - Pat the salmon filets dry with paper towels and place them on a baking sheet lined with parchment paper.
    - Drizzle olive oil over the salmon filets and season with salt and pepper.
    - In a small bowl, mix together the chopped dill, lemon juice, minced garlic, and Greek yogurt to make the lemon dill sauce.
    - Spread a spoonful of the lemon dill sauce over each salmon filet, covering them evenly.
3. Roast the asparagus:
    - Place the trimmed asparagus on another baking sheet lined with parchment paper.
    - Drizzle olive oil over the asparagus and season with salt and pepper. Toss to coat evenly.
    - Optional: sprinkle lemon zest over the asparagus for extra flavor.
    - Place both the salmon and asparagus in the preheated oven.
4. Roast for 12-15 minutes, or until the salmon is cooked through and flakes easily with a fork, and the asparagus is tender yet crisp.

5. Serve the roasted salmon with lemon wedges on the side and garnish with additional chopped dill, if desired. Serve the roasted asparagus alongside.

Chicken Stir-Fry with Brown Rice and Vegetables

Ingredients:

- 2 boneless, skinless chicken breasts, thinly sliced
- 2 tablespoons low-sodium soy sauce
- 1 tablespoon rice vinegar
- 1 tablespoon honey or maple syrup
- 2 cloves garlic, minced
- 1 teaspoon grated fresh ginger
- 1 tablespoon olive oil or sesame oil
- 4 cups mixed vegetables (such as bell peppers, broccoli, carrots, snap peas)
- Cooked brown rice for serving
- Optional garnish: sliced green onions, sesame seeds

Directions:

1. In a small bowl, whisk together soy sauce, rice vinegar, honey or maple syrup, minced garlic, and grated ginger to make the stir-fry sauce. Set aside.

2. Heat olive oil or sesame oil in a large skillet or wok over medium-high heat. Add the sliced chicken breasts and cook until browned and cooked through, about 5-7 minutes. Remove the chicken from the skillet and set aside.

3. In the same skillet, add the mixed vegetables and stir-fry for 3-5 minutes, or until they are tender yet still crisp.

4. Return the cooked chicken to the skillet and pour the stir-fry sauce over the chicken and vegetables. Stir well to coat everything evenly with the sauce.

5. Cook for an additional 2-3 minutes, or until the sauce has thickened slightly and everything is heated through.

6. Serve the chicken stir-fry hot over cooked brown rice. Garnish with sliced green onions and sesame seeds if desired.

Turkey Taco Bowls with Low-Carb Tortillas or Lettuce Wraps

Ingredients:

- 1 lb lean ground turkey
- 1 tablespoon olive oil
- 1 small onion, diced
- 2 cloves garlic, minced
- 1 bell pepper, diced
- 1 tablespoon chili powder
- 1 teaspoon ground cumin
- 1/2 teaspoon paprika
- 1/4 teaspoon cayenne pepper (optional, for heat)
- Salt and pepper to taste
- 1 cup cooked brown rice or cauliflower rice
- 1 cup black beans, drained and rinsed
- 1 cup diced tomatoes
- 1 cup shredded lettuce
- 1/2 cup shredded cheese (optional)
- Sliced avocado for garnish

- Fresh cilantro for garnish
- Low-carb tortillas or lettuce wraps for serving

Directions:

1. Heat olive oil in a large skillet over medium heat. Add diced onion and cook until softened, about 3-4 minutes.
2. Add minced garlic and diced bell pepper to the skillet. Cook for another 2-3 minutes, until the bell pepper is tender.
3. Add ground turkey to the skillet, breaking it apart with a spatula. Cook until browned and cooked through, about 5-7 minutes.
4. Stir in chili powder, ground cumin, paprika, cayenne pepper (if using), salt, and pepper. Cook for another minute to toast the spices.
5. Add cooked brown rice or cauliflower rice, black beans, and diced tomatoes to the skillet. Stir to combine and cook until heated through, about 2-3 minutes.
6. Remove the skillet from heat. Assemble the taco bowls by dividing the turkey mixture among serving bowls.
7. Top each bowl with shredded lettuce, shredded cheese (if using), sliced avocado, and fresh cilantro.
8. Serve the turkey taco bowls with low-carb tortillas or lettuce wraps on the side for wrapping or scooping.

One-Pan Lemon Garlic Shrimp with Roasted Vegetables

One-Pan Lemon Garlic Shrimp:

Ingredients:

- 1 lb large shrimp, peeled and deveined
- 2 tablespoons olive oil

- 4 cloves garlic, minced
- Zest and juice of 1 lemon
- 1 teaspoon dried oregano
- Salt and pepper to taste
- Lemon slices for garnish
- Chopped fresh parsley for garnish

Roasted Vegetables:

Ingredients:

- 2 cups mixed vegetables (such as bell peppers, zucchini, cherry tomatoes, broccoli florets)
- 1 tablespoon olive oil
- Salt and pepper to taste
- Optional: additional minced garlic, dried herbs (such as thyme or rosemary)

Directions:

1. Preheat your oven to 400°F (200°C).
2. In a large bowl, combine the peeled and deveined shrimp with olive oil, minced garlic, lemon zest, lemon juice, dried oregano, salt, and pepper. Toss to coat the shrimp evenly with the seasoning.
3. Spread the seasoned shrimp in a single layer on a baking sheet lined with parchment paper or aluminum foil. Arrange lemon slices on top of the shrimp for extra flavor.
4. In the same bowl used for the shrimp, toss the mixed vegetables with olive oil, salt, pepper, minced garlic (if using), and dried herbs (if using).
5. Spread the seasoned vegetables in a single layer on another baking sheet lined with parchment paper or aluminum foil.

6. Place both the shrimp and vegetables in the preheated oven. Roast for 10-12 minutes, or until the shrimp are pink and cooked through, and the vegetables are tender and slightly caramelized around the edges.

7. Remove the baking sheets from the oven. Sprinkle chopped fresh parsley over the roasted shrimp for garnish.

8. Serve the One-Pan Lemon Garlic Shrimp with Roasted Vegetables hot, garnished with additional lemon slices if desired.

Lentil Shepherd's Pie with Mashed Cauliflower

Lentil Shepherd's Pie:

Ingredients:

- 1 cup dry green or brown lentils
- 2 cups vegetable broth
- 1 tablespoon olive oil
- 1 onion, diced
- 2 carrots, diced
- 2 celery stalks, diced
- 2 cloves garlic, minced
- 1 teaspoon dried thyme
- 1 teaspoon dried rosemary
- 1 cup frozen peas
- Salt and pepper to taste
- Mashed cauliflower (see recipe below)

Mashed Cauliflower:

Ingredients:

- 1 large head cauliflower, cut into florets
- 2 cloves garlic, minced

- 2 tablespoons unsweetened almond milk or low-fat milk
- 1 tablespoon olive oil or butter
- Salt and pepper to taste

Directions:

1. Preheat your oven to 375°F (190°C).

2. Rinse the lentils under cold water and drain them. In a saucepan, combine the lentils and vegetable broth. Bring to a boil, then reduce heat and simmer for about 20-25 minutes, or until the lentils are tender and most of the liquid is absorbed.

3. While the lentils are cooking, prepare the mashed cauliflower. Steam the cauliflower florets until tender, about 10-12 minutes. Drain well.

4. In a large mixing bowl, mash the cooked cauliflower with a potato masher or fork until smooth. Stir in minced garlic, almond milk or low-fat milk, olive oil or butter, salt, and pepper. Set aside.

5. In a large skillet, heat olive oil over medium heat. Add diced onion, carrots, and celery. Cook until vegetables are softened, about 5-7 minutes.

6. Add minced garlic, dried thyme, and dried rosemary to the skillet. Cook for another 1-2 minutes until fragrant.

7. Stir in cooked lentils and frozen peas. Season with salt and pepper to taste. Cook for an additional 2-3 minutes to heat everything through.

8. Transfer the lentil and vegetable mixture to a baking dish. Spread the mashed cauliflower evenly over the top.

9. Bake in the preheated oven for 25-30 minutes, or until the mashed cauliflower is lightly golden on top.

10. Remove from the oven and let it cool slightly before serving.

11. Serve your Lentil Shepherd's Pie with Mashed Cauliflower hot, and enjoy this comforting and nutritious meal!

Black Bean Burgers on Whole-Wheat Buns with Sweet Potato Fries

Black Bean Burgers:

Ingredients:

- 2 cans (15 ounces each) black beans, drained and rinsed
- 1/2 cup finely diced onion
- 1/2 cup finely diced bell pepper (any color)
- 2 cloves garlic, minced
- 1 teaspoon ground cumin
- 1 teaspoon chili powder
- 1/2 teaspoon smoked paprika
- 1/4 teaspoon cayenne pepper (optional, for heat)
- 1/4 cup chopped fresh cilantro
- 1/2 cup breadcrumbs (whole-wheat or gluten-free)
- 1 egg, beaten
- Salt and pepper to taste
- Olive oil for cooking

For serving:

- Whole-wheat burger buns
- Lettuce leaves
- Sliced tomatoes
- Sliced red onion
- Avocado slices
- Mustard or your favorite burger condiments

Sweet Potato Fries:

Ingredients:

- 2 large sweet potatoes, peeled and cut into fries
- 2 tablespoons olive oil
- 1 teaspoon smoked paprika
- 1/2 teaspoon garlic powder
- 1/2 teaspoon onion powder
- Salt and pepper to taste

Directions:

1. Preheat your oven to 425°F (220°C).
2. In a large mixing bowl, mash the black beans with a fork or potato masher until mostly smooth but still slightly chunky.
3. Add diced onion, diced bell pepper, minced garlic, ground cumin, chili powder, smoked paprika, cayenne pepper (if using), chopped cilantro, breadcrumbs, beaten egg, salt, and pepper to the bowl. Mix until everything is well combined.
4. Divide the black bean mixture into 4 equal portions and shape them into burger patties.
5. Heat a tablespoon of olive oil in a skillet over medium heat. Cook the black bean burgers for about 4-5 minutes on each side, or until they are golden brown and heated through. Alternatively, you can bake the burgers in the oven at 375°F (190°C) for 20-25 minutes, flipping halfway through.
6. While the burgers are cooking, prepare the sweet potato fries. In a large bowl, toss the sweet potato fries with olive oil, smoked paprika, garlic powder, onion powder, salt, and pepper until evenly coated.

7. Arrange the sweet potato fries in a single layer on a baking sheet lined with parchment paper. Bake in the preheated oven for 20-25 minutes, or until the fries are crispy and golden brown, flipping halfway through.

8. Toast the whole-wheat burger buns if desired. Assemble the black bean burgers on the buns with lettuce leaves, sliced tomatoes, sliced red onion, avocado slices, and your favorite burger condiments.

9. Serve the black bean burgers with sweet potato fries on the side.

Baked Chicken Fajitas with Whole-Wheat Tortillas and Grilled Vegetables

Baked Chicken Fajitas:

Ingredients:

- 1 lb boneless, skinless chicken breasts, thinly sliced
- 2 bell peppers (any color), thinly sliced
- 1 onion, thinly sliced
- 2 tablespoons olive oil
- 1 tablespoon chili powder
- 1 teaspoon ground cumin
- 1/2 teaspoon smoked paprika
- 1/2 teaspoon garlic powder
- 1/2 teaspoon onion powder
- Salt and pepper to taste
- Whole-wheat tortillas for serving
- Optional toppings: sliced avocado, shredded lettuce, diced tomatoes, Greek yogurt or sour cream, shredded cheese, salsa

Grilled Vegetables:

Ingredients:

- 2 zucchini, sliced lengthwise
- 2 yellow squash, sliced lengthwise
- 1 red onion, sliced into rounds
- 1 tablespoon olive oil
- Salt and pepper to taste

Directions:

1. Preheat your oven to 400°F (200°C).
2. In a large mixing bowl, combine the sliced chicken breasts, sliced bell peppers, sliced onion, olive oil, chili powder, ground cumin, smoked paprika, garlic powder, onion powder, salt, and pepper. Toss until everything is well coated.
3. Transfer the chicken and vegetable mixture to a large baking sheet lined with parchment paper or aluminum foil, spreading it out evenly.
4. Bake in the preheated oven for 20-25 minutes, or until the chicken is cooked through and the vegetables are tender and slightly caramelized around the edges.
5. While the chicken fajitas are baking, prepare the grilled vegetables. Preheat a grill pan or outdoor grill over medium-high heat.
6. In a large bowl, toss the sliced zucchini, yellow squash, and red onion with olive oil, salt, and pepper until evenly coated.
7. Grill the vegetables for 3-4 minutes on each side, or until they are tender and have grill marks.
8. Once the chicken fajitas and grilled vegetables are cooked, remove them from the oven and grill, respectively.

9. Serve the baked chicken fajitas and grilled vegetables with warm whole-wheat tortillas and optional toppings such as sliced avocado, shredded lettuce, diced tomatoes, Greek yogurt or sour cream, shredded cheese, and salsa.

Salmon with Roasted Brussels Sprouts and Quinoa

Salmon:

Ingredients:

- 4 salmon filets (about 4-6 ounces each)
- 2 tablespoons olive oil
- 2 cloves garlic, minced
- 1 teaspoon dried thyme
- 1 teaspoon dried rosemary
- Salt and pepper to taste
- Lemon wedges for serving

Roasted Brussels Sprouts:

Ingredients:

- 1 lb Brussels sprouts, trimmed and halved
- 2 tablespoons olive oil
- 2 cloves garlic, minced
- Salt and pepper to taste

Quinoa:

Ingredients:

- 1 cup quinoa, rinsed
- 2 cups vegetable broth or water
- Salt to taste

Directions:

1. Preheat your oven to 400°F (200°C).

2. In a small bowl, mix together olive oil, minced garlic, dried thyme, dried rosemary, salt, and pepper. Brush the mixture over the salmon filets.

3. Place the salmon filets on a baking sheet lined with parchment paper or aluminum foil. Bake in the preheated oven for 12-15 minutes, or until the salmon is cooked through and flakes easily with a fork.

4. While the salmon is baking, prepare the roasted Brussels sprouts. In a large mixing bowl, toss the halved Brussels sprouts with olive oil, minced garlic, salt, and pepper until evenly coated.

5. Spread the Brussels sprouts in a single layer on another baking sheet lined with parchment paper or aluminum foil. Roast in the preheated oven for 20-25 minutes, or until they are tender and caramelized around the edges.

6. While the salmon and Brussels sprouts are cooking, prepare the quinoa. In a medium saucepan, combine quinoa and vegetable broth or water. Bring to a boil, then reduce heat to low, cover, and simmer for 15-20 minutes, or until the quinoa is cooked and liquid is absorbed. Fluff with a fork and season with salt to taste.

7. Once everything is cooked, divide the quinoa among serving plates. Top with roasted Brussels sprouts and baked salmon filets. Serve with lemon wedges on the side for squeezing over the salmon.

8. Enjoy your delicious and nutritious Salmon with Roasted Brussels Sprouts and Quinoa!

Chicken and Vegetable Curry with Brown Rice

Chicken and Vegetable Curry:

Ingredients:

- 1 lb boneless, skinless chicken breasts or thighs, cut into bite-sized pieces
- 2 tablespoons olive oil or coconut oil
- 1 onion, chopped
- 2 cloves garlic, minced
- 1 tablespoon fresh ginger, minced
- 1 bell pepper, chopped
- 1 zucchini, chopped
- 1 cup chopped carrots
- 1 cup chopped cauliflower florets
- 1 cup chopped green beans
- 2 tablespoons curry powder
- 1 teaspoon ground turmeric
- 1 teaspoon ground cumin
- 1 teaspoon ground coriander
- 1 can (14 ounces) coconut milk
- 1 cup vegetable broth
- Salt and pepper to taste
- Fresh cilantro for garnish

Brown Rice:

Ingredients:

- 1 cup brown rice
- 2 cups water or vegetable broth
- Salt to taste

Directions:

1. In a large skillet or Dutch oven, heat olive oil or coconut oil over medium heat. Add chopped onion and cook until softened, about 5 minutes.

2. Add minced garlic and minced ginger to the skillet. Cook for another 1-2 minutes until fragrant.

3. Add chicken pieces to the skillet and cook until browned on all sides, about 5-7 minutes.

4. Stir in chopped bell pepper, zucchini, carrots, cauliflower florets, and green beans. Cook for another 5 minutes, stirring occasionally.

5. Sprinkle curry powder, ground turmeric, ground cumin, and ground coriander over the chicken and vegetables. Stir well to coat everything evenly with the spices.

6. Pour in coconut milk and vegetable broth. Stir to combine.

7. Bring the curry to a simmer, then reduce heat to low and cover. Let it simmer gently for 20-25 minutes, or until the chicken is cooked through and the vegetables are tender.

8. While the curry is simmering, prepare the brown rice. In a medium saucepan, combine brown rice and water or vegetable broth. Bring to a boil, then reduce heat to low, cover, and simmer for 40-45 minutes, or until the rice is tender and liquid is absorbed. Fluff with a fork and season with salt to taste.

9. Once the curry is ready, taste and adjust seasoning with salt and pepper as needed.

10. Serve the Chicken and Vegetable Curry hot over cooked brown rice. Garnish with fresh cilantro leaves.

11. Enjoy your delicious and nutritious Chicken and Vegetable Curry with Brown Rice!

Tofu Scramble with Whole-Wheat Toast and Avocado

Tofu Scramble:

Ingredients:

- 1 block (14 ounces) firm tofu, drained and pressed
- 2 tablespoons olive oil
- 1 small onion, diced
- 1 bell pepper, diced
- 2 cloves garlic, minced
- 1 teaspoon ground turmeric
- 1/2 teaspoon ground cumin
- 1/2 teaspoon chili powder
- Salt and pepper to taste
- 2 tablespoons nutritional yeast (optional, for a cheesy flavor)
- Fresh parsley or cilantro for garnish (optional)

Whole-Wheat Toast and Avocado:

Ingredients:

- Whole-wheat bread slices
- 1 ripe avocado, sliced
- Salt and pepper to taste

Directions:

1. Start by preparing the tofu scramble. In a large skillet, heat olive oil over medium heat. Add diced onion and bell pepper. Cook until softened, about 5 minutes.

2. Crumble the pressed tofu into the skillet using your hands or a fork. Cook for another 5-7 minutes, stirring occasionally, until the tofu starts to brown slightly.

3. Add minced garlic, ground turmeric, ground cumin, chili powder, salt, and pepper to the skillet. Stir well to coat the tofu and vegetables evenly with the spices. Cook for another 2-3 minutes, until the garlic is fragrant and the spices are toasted.

4. Optional: Sprinkle nutritional yeast over the tofu scramble for a cheesy flavor. Stir to combine.

5. While the tofu scramble is cooking, toast the whole-wheat bread slices until golden brown.

6. Once the tofu scramble is ready, remove from heat and garnish with fresh parsley or cilantro if desired.

7. To assemble, spread sliced avocado on top of the toasted whole-wheat bread slices. Season with salt and pepper to taste.

8. Serve the Tofu Scramble with Whole-Wheat Toast and Avocado hot, and enjoy this nutritious and satisfying meal!

Tuna Noodle Casserole with Whole-Wheat Noodles and Light Cream Sauce

Ingredients:

- 8 ounces whole-wheat egg noodles
- 2 cans (5 ounces each) tuna in water, drained
- 2 cups frozen peas and carrots, thawed
- 1 tablespoon olive oil
- 1 onion, diced
- 2 cloves garlic, minced

- 2 tablespoons whole wheat flour
- 1 1/2 cups low-fat milk
- 1/2 cup low-sodium chicken or vegetable broth
- 1/2 teaspoon dried thyme
- 1/2 teaspoon dried parsley
- Salt and pepper to taste
- 1/4 cup grated Parmesan cheese
- 1/4 cup whole-wheat breadcrumbs
- Cooking spray

Directions:

1. Preheat your oven to 375°F (190°C). Lightly grease a 9x13-inch baking dish with cooking spray.
2. Cook the whole-wheat egg noodles according to the package instructions until al dente. Drain and set aside.
3. In a large skillet, heat olive oil over medium heat. Add diced onion and cook until softened, about 5 minutes. Add minced garlic and cook for another 1-2 minutes until fragrant.
4. Sprinkle whole wheat flour over the onion and garlic mixture. Stir well to coat the flour evenly.
5. Slowly pour in low-fat milk and low-sodium chicken or vegetable broth, stirring constantly to prevent lumps from forming. Cook until the sauce thickens, about 5 minutes.
6. Stir in dried thyme, dried parsley, salt, and pepper to taste.
7. Add drained tuna, thawed peas and carrots, and cooked whole-wheat egg noodles to the skillet. Stir until everything is well combined and coated with the cream sauce.

8. Transfer the tuna noodle mixture to the prepared baking dish and spread it out evenly.

9. In a small bowl, combine grated Parmesan cheese and whole-wheat breadcrumbs. Sprinkle the breadcrumb mixture evenly over the top of the casserole.

10. Lightly spray the breadcrumb topping with cooking spray to help it brown.

11. Bake in the preheated oven for 20-25 minutes, or until the casserole is heated through and the topping is golden brown and crispy.

12. Remove from the oven and let it cool for a few minutes before serving.

13. Serve your Tuna Noodle Casserole with Whole-Wheat Noodles and Light Cream Sauce hot, and enjoy this nutritious and comforting meal!

Chicken Souvlaki Bowls with Lemon Herb Marinade and Whole-Wheat Pita Bread

Chicken Souvlaki:

Ingredients:

- 1 lb boneless, skinless chicken breasts, cut into bite-sized pieces
- 2 tablespoons olive oil
- 2 cloves garlic, minced
- Juice and zest of 1 lemon
- 1 teaspoon dried oregano
- 1 teaspoon dried thyme
- 1 teaspoon dried rosemary
- Salt and pepper to taste

Lemon Herb Marinade:

Ingredients:

- Juice and zest of 1 lemon
- 2 tablespoons olive oil
- 2 cloves garlic, minced
- 1 teaspoon dried oregano
- 1 teaspoon dried thyme
- 1 teaspoon dried rosemary
- Salt and pepper to taste

For serving:

- Cooked quinoa or brown rice
- Chopped lettuce or mixed greens
- Sliced cucumber
- Sliced tomatoes
- Sliced red onion
- Whole-wheat pita bread

Directions:

1. In a large mixing bowl, combine olive oil, minced garlic, lemon zest, lemon juice, dried oregano, dried thyme, dried rosemary, salt, and pepper. Stir well to make the marinade.
2. Add the chicken pieces to the marinade and toss until evenly coated. Cover the bowl and refrigerate for at least 30 minutes, or up to 2 hours, to marinate.
3. While the chicken is marinating, prepare the Lemon Herb Marinade. In a small bowl, combine lemon juice, lemon zest, olive oil, minced garlic, dried oregano, dried thyme, dried rosemary, salt, and pepper. Stir well to combine.

4. Preheat your grill or grill pan over medium-high heat. Thread the marinated chicken pieces onto skewers.

5. Grill the chicken skewers for 5-7 minutes per side, or until the chicken is cooked through and has grill marks. Remove from the grill and let it rest for a few minutes.

6. While the chicken is resting, prepare the serving bowls. Divide cooked quinoa or brown rice, chopped lettuce or mixed greens, sliced cucumber, sliced tomatoes, and sliced red onion among serving bowls.

7. Remove the chicken from the skewers and add it to the serving bowls.

8. Drizzle the Lemon Herb Marinade over the chicken and vegetables in the bowls.

9. Serve the Chicken Souvlaki Bowls with Lemon Herb Marinade with whole-wheat pita bread on the side.

Vegetarian Chili with Kidney Beans and Corn

Ingredients:
- 2 tablespoons olive oil
- 1 onion, diced
- 2 cloves garlic, minced
- 1 bell pepper, diced (any color)
- 1 zucchini, diced
- 1 carrot, diced
- 1 jalapeño pepper, seeded and diced (optional, for heat)
- 1 can (14 ounces) diced tomatoes
- 1 can (14 ounces) tomato sauce
- 2 cans (14 ounces each) kidney beans, drained and rinsed
- 1 cup frozen corn kernels

- 2 tablespoons chili powder

- 1 teaspoon ground cumin

- 1 teaspoon paprika

- Salt and pepper to taste

- Optional toppings: shredded cheese, diced avocado, chopped cilantro, Greek yogurt or sour cream

Directions:

1. In a large pot or Dutch oven, heat olive oil over medium heat. Add diced onion and cook until softened, about 5 minutes.

2. Add minced garlic and diced bell pepper to the pot. Cook for another 2-3 minutes until fragrant.

3. Stir in diced zucchini, diced carrot, and diced jalapeño pepper (if using). Cook for another 5 minutes, stirring occasionally.

4. Add diced tomatoes, tomato sauce, kidney beans, frozen corn kernels, chili powder, ground cumin, paprika, salt, and pepper to the pot. Stir well to combine.

5. Bring the chili to a simmer, then reduce heat to low. Cover and let it simmer for 20-30 minutes, stirring occasionally, to allow the flavors to meld and the vegetables to soften.

6. Taste and adjust seasoning with additional salt and pepper if needed.

7. Once the chili is ready, ladle it into bowls and serve hot.

8. Garnish each serving with your choice of toppings, such as shredded cheese, diced avocado, chopped cilantro, and Greek yogurt or sour cream.

9. Enjoy your delicious and nutritious Vegetarian Chili with Kidney Beans and Corn!

Baked Cod with Lemon and Herbs and Roasted Vegetables

Baked Cod with Lemon and Herbs:

Ingredients:

- 4 cod filets (about 6 ounces each)
- 2 tablespoons olive oil
- 2 cloves garlic, minced
- Zest and juice of 1 lemon
- 1 teaspoon dried thyme
- 1 teaspoon dried parsley
- Salt and pepper to taste
- Lemon slices for garnish
- Fresh parsley for garnish (optional)

Roasted Vegetables:

Ingredients:

- 2 cups mixed vegetables (such as bell peppers, zucchini, cherry tomatoes, and red onion), chopped
- 2 tablespoons olive oil
- Salt and pepper to taste

Directions:

1. Preheat your oven to 400°F (200°C). Line a baking sheet with parchment paper or aluminum foil.
2. In a small bowl, whisk together olive oil, minced garlic, lemon zest, lemon juice, dried thyme, dried parsley, salt, and pepper.
3. Place the cod filets on the prepared baking sheet. Brush the lemon and herb mixture over the top of each filet, coating them evenly.

4. Arrange lemon slices on top of each cod filet for extra flavor. You can also sprinkle fresh parsley over the top for added garnish if desired.

5. Transfer the baking sheet to the preheated oven and bake for 12-15 minutes, or until the cod is opaque and flakes easily with a fork.

6. While the cod is baking, prepare the roasted vegetables. In a large mixing bowl, toss the chopped mixed vegetables with olive oil, salt, and pepper until evenly coated.

7. Spread the seasoned vegetables out in a single layer on another baking sheet lined with parchment paper or aluminum foil.

8. Place the baking sheet with the vegetables in the oven alongside the cod during the last 10-15 minutes of baking, or until the vegetables are tender and slightly caramelized around the edges.

9. Once the cod and roasted vegetables are cooked, remove them from the oven.

10. Serve the Baked Cod with Lemon and Herbs alongside the Roasted Vegetables.

Chicken and Vegetable Sheet-Pan Dinner

Ingredients:

- 4 boneless, skinless chicken breasts
- 2 bell peppers (any color), sliced
- 1 red onion, sliced
- 1 zucchini, sliced
- 1 yellow squash, sliced
- 1 cup cherry tomatoes
- 2 tablespoons olive oil
- 2 cloves garlic, minced

- 1 teaspoon dried thyme
- 1 teaspoon dried rosemary
- 1 teaspoon dried oregano
- Salt and pepper to taste
- Fresh parsley for garnish (optional)

Directions:

1. Preheat your oven to 400°F (200°C). Line a large baking sheet with parchment paper or aluminum foil for easy cleanup.
2. Place the chicken breasts in the center of the baking sheet, leaving some space around them for the vegetables.
3. In a small bowl, whisk together olive oil, minced garlic, dried thyme, dried rosemary, dried oregano, salt, and pepper.
4. Brush the olive oil mixture over the chicken breasts, coating them evenly.
5. Arrange the sliced bell peppers, red onion, zucchini, yellow squash, and cherry tomatoes around the chicken on the baking sheet.
6. Drizzle any remaining olive oil mixture over the vegetables.
7. Transfer the baking sheet to the preheated oven and bake for 20-25 minutes, or until the chicken is cooked through and the vegetables are tender and slightly caramelized around the edges.
8. Once the chicken and vegetables are cooked, remove the baking sheet from the oven.
9. Garnish with fresh parsley if desired.
10. Serve your Chicken and Vegetable Sheet-Pan Dinner hot, and enjoy this delicious and nutritious meal!

Turkey Meatloaf with Mashed Sweet Potatoes

Turkey Meatloaf:

Ingredients:

- 1 lb ground turkey
- 1/2 cup breadcrumbs (preferably whole wheat)
- 1/4 cup grated Parmesan cheese
- 1 small onion, finely chopped
- 2 cloves garlic, minced
- 1/4 cup ketchup or tomato sauce
- 1 tablespoon Worcestershire sauce
- 1 teaspoon dried thyme
- 1 teaspoon dried oregano
- 1/2 teaspoon paprika
- Salt and pepper to taste
- Cooking spray

Mashed Sweet Potatoes:

Ingredients:

- 2 large sweet potatoes, peeled and diced
- 2 tablespoons unsalted butter or olive oil
- 1/4 cup milk (any type, dairy or non-dairy)
- Salt and pepper to taste

Directions:

1. Preheat your oven to 375°F (190°C). Lightly grease a loaf pan with cooking spray.

2. In a large mixing bowl, combine ground turkey, breadcrumbs, grated Parmesan cheese, finely chopped onion, minced garlic, ketchup or tomato sauce, Worcestershire sauce, dried thyme, dried oregano, paprika, salt, and pepper. Mix until well combined.

3. Transfer the turkey mixture to the prepared loaf pan, pressing it down evenly.

4. Bake the meatloaf in the preheated oven for 45-50 minutes, or until cooked through and browned on top. Make sure the internal temperature of the meatloaf reaches 165°F (75°C) for safe consumption.

5. While the meatloaf is baking, prepare the mashed sweet potatoes. Place the diced sweet potatoes in a large pot and cover them with water. Bring to a boil over medium-high heat, then reduce the heat to medium-low and simmer for 15-20 minutes, or until the sweet potatoes are tender when pierced with a fork.

6. Drain the cooked sweet potatoes and return them to the pot. Add unsalted butter or olive oil, milk, salt, and pepper to taste.

7. Mash the sweet potatoes with a potato masher or fork until smooth and creamy. Adjust the seasoning if needed.

8. Once the meatloaf is done baking, remove it from the oven and let it rest for a few minutes before slicing.

9. Serve slices of Turkey Meatloaf with a generous serving of Mashed Sweet Potatoes.

10. Enjoy your delicious and nutritious Turkey Meatloaf with Mashed Sweet Potatoes!

Shrimp Scampi with Zucchini Noodles and Whole-Wheat Toast

Ingredients:

- 1 lb large shrimp, peeled and deveined
- 3 medium zucchini
- 4 cloves garlic, minced
- 2 tablespoons olive oil
- 1/4 cup white wine (optional)
- Juice of 1 lemon
- 2 tablespoons unsalted butter
- Salt and pepper to taste
- Crushed red pepper flakes (optional)
- Chopped fresh parsley for garnish
- 4 slices whole-wheat bread

Directions:

1. Using a spiralizer, spiralize the zucchini into noodles. Alternatively, you can use a vegetable peeler to make zucchini ribbons.
2. Heat 1 tablespoon of olive oil in a large skillet over medium heat. Add the shrimp and cook for 2-3 minutes per side, or until they turn pink and opaque. Remove the shrimp from the skillet and set aside.
3. In the same skillet, add the remaining tablespoon of olive oil. Add the minced garlic and cook for 1-2 minutes, or until fragrant.
4. If using white wine, add it to the skillet and let it simmer for 1-2 minutes, allowing the alcohol to evaporate.

5. Add the zucchini noodles to the skillet and toss to coat them in the garlic and olive oil mixture. Cook for 2-3 minutes, or until the zucchini noodles are just tender. Be careful not to overcook them, as they can become mushy.

6. Return the cooked shrimp to the skillet. Add the lemon juice and unsalted butter. Season with salt, pepper, and crushed red pepper flakes to taste. Toss everything together until the shrimp are heated through and the butter is melted.

7. While the shrimp scampi is cooking, toast the whole-wheat bread slices until golden brown.

8. Divide the shrimp scampi and zucchini noodles among serving plates. Garnish with chopped fresh parsley.

9. Serve the Shrimp Scampi with Zucchini Noodles alongside the whole-wheat toast.

Chicken Breast with Mango Salsa and Black Beans

Ingredients:

For the Chicken:

- 4 boneless, skinless chicken breasts
- 2 tablespoons olive oil
- 1 teaspoon ground cumin
- 1 teaspoon paprika
- Salt and pepper to taste

For the Mango Salsa:

- 2 ripe mangoes, peeled, pitted, and diced
- 1/2 red onion, finely chopped
- 1 jalapeño pepper, seeded and finely chopped

- Juice of 1 lime

- 2 tablespoons chopped fresh cilantro

- Salt to taste

For the Black Beans:

- 1 can (15 ounces) black beans, drained and rinsed

- 1 clove garlic, minced

- 1 teaspoon ground cumin

- 1/2 teaspoon chili powder

- Salt and pepper to taste

Directions:

1. Preheat your grill or grill pan over medium-high heat.

2. In a small bowl, mix together olive oil, ground cumin, paprika, salt, and pepper. Brush the mixture over both sides of the chicken breasts.

3. Grill the chicken breasts for 6-7 minutes per side, or until they are cooked through and have grill marks. The internal temperature of the chicken should reach 165°F (75°C). Remove the chicken from the grill and let it rest for a few minutes.

4. While the chicken is grilling, prepare the mango salsa. In a medium bowl, combine diced mangoes, finely chopped red onion, finely chopped jalapeño pepper, lime juice, chopped fresh cilantro, and salt to taste. Stir well to combine. Set aside.

5. In a small saucepan, heat a bit of olive oil over medium heat. Add minced garlic and cook for 1 minute, or until fragrant.

6. Add drained and rinsed black beans to the saucepan, along with ground cumin, chili powder, salt, and pepper. Cook for 3-4 minutes, stirring occasionally, until the beans are heated through and well seasoned.

7. Once the chicken breasts have rested, slice them thinly.

8. To serve, place a portion of sliced chicken breast on each plate. Top with a generous spoonful of mango salsa and a side of seasoned black beans.

9. Enjoy your flavorful and nutritious Chicken Breast with Mango Salsa and Black Beans!

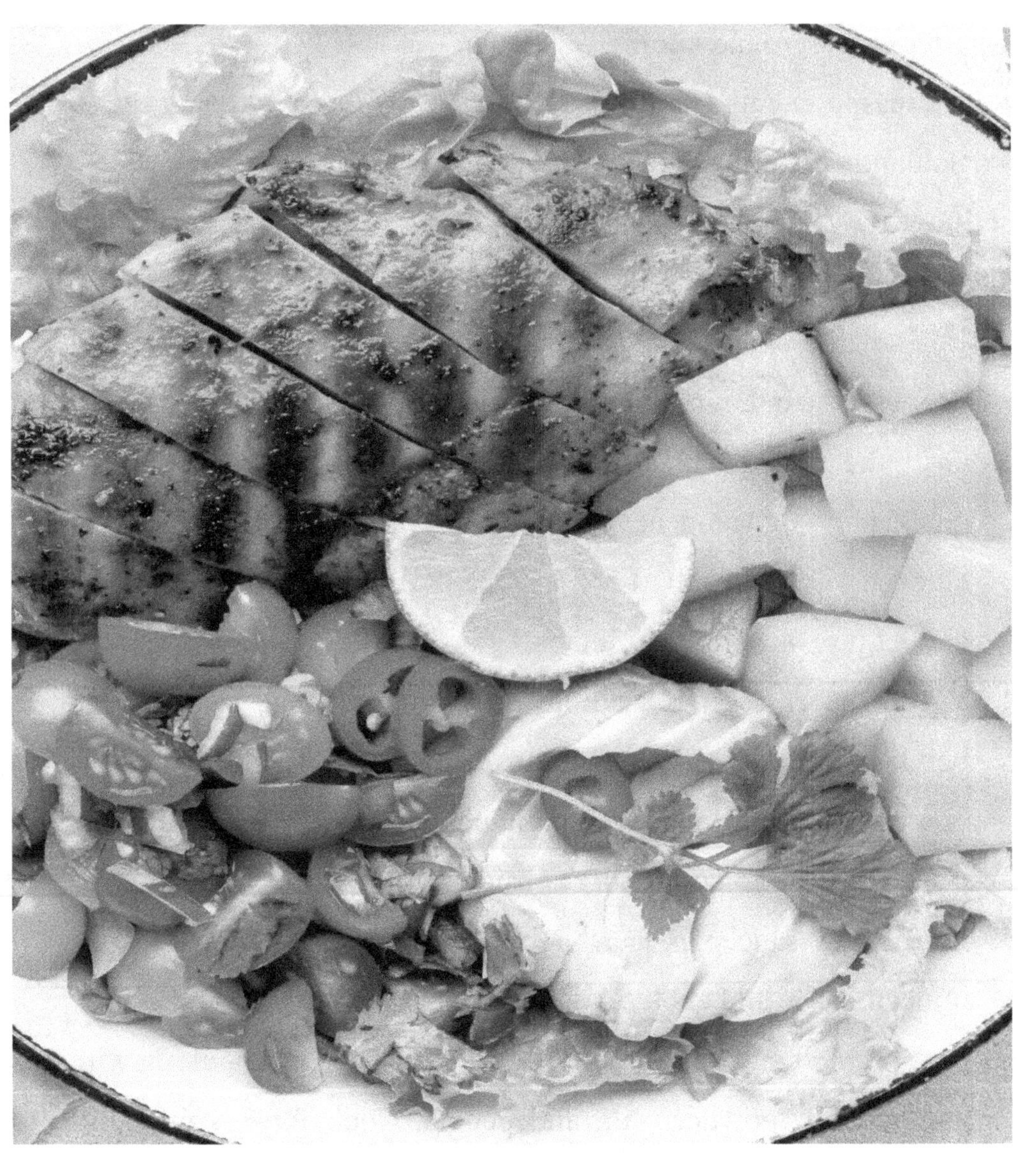

Chapter 8: Fish and Seafood Recipes

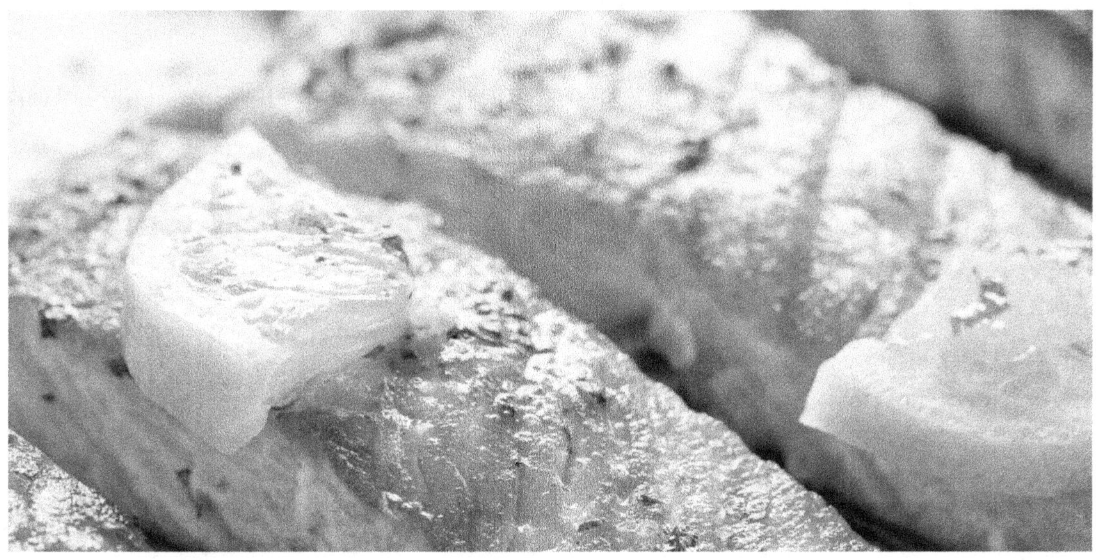

Baked Tilapia with Lemon Herb Crust and Roasted Asparagus

Ingredients:

For the Baked Tilapia:

- 4 tilapia filets (about 6 ounces each)
- 2 tablespoons olive oil
- Zest of 1 lemon
- 2 cloves garlic, minced
- 1 teaspoon dried thyme
- 1 teaspoon dried parsley
- Salt and pepper to taste
- Lemon slices for garnish

For the Roasted Asparagus:

- 1 bunch asparagus, woody ends trimmed

- 1 tablespoon olive oil
- Salt and pepper to taste

Directions:

1. Preheat your oven to 400°F (200°C). Line a baking sheet with parchment paper.
2. In a small bowl, mix together olive oil, lemon zest, minced garlic, dried thyme, dried parsley, salt, and pepper to create the lemon herb crust.
3. Place the tilapia filets on the prepared baking sheet. Brush the lemon herb crust mixture evenly over each filet.
4. Place a lemon slice on top of each filet for added flavor.
5. Arrange the trimmed asparagus on the same baking sheet, drizzle with olive oil, and season with salt and pepper.
6. Transfer the baking sheet to the preheated oven and bake for 12-15 minutes, or until the tilapia is cooked through and flakes easily with a fork, and the asparagus is tender.
7. Once the tilapia and asparagus are done baking, remove them from the oven.
8. Serve the Baked Tilapia with Lemon Herb Crust alongside the Roasted Asparagus.

Cajun Shrimp with Veggie Grits

Ingredients:

For the Cajun Shrimp:

- 1 lb large shrimp, peeled and deveined
- 2 tablespoons Cajun seasoning
- 2 tablespoons olive oil
- 2 cloves garlic, minced

- Juice of 1 lemon

- Salt and pepper to taste

- Chopped fresh parsley for garnish

For the Veggie Grits:

- 1 cup stone-ground grits

- 3 cups water or low-sodium chicken broth

- 1 tablespoon olive oil

- 1 small onion, diced

- 1 bell pepper, diced

- 1 zucchini, diced

- 1 cup cherry tomatoes, halved

- Salt and pepper to taste

- Optional: grated cheese for serving

Directions:

1. In a large bowl, toss the shrimp with Cajun seasoning, minced garlic, olive oil, lemon juice, salt, and pepper until evenly coated. Let marinate for at least 15 minutes.

2. Meanwhile, prepare the veggie grits. In a medium saucepan, bring water or chicken broth to a boil. Stir in the stone-ground grits and reduce the heat to low. Cook, stirring occasionally, for about 20-25 minutes, or until the grits are creamy and tender.

3. While the grits are cooking, heat 1 tablespoon of olive oil in a large skillet over medium heat. Add diced onion and bell pepper, and sauté for 3-4 minutes, until softened.

4. Add diced zucchini to the skillet and cook for another 2-3 minutes, until slightly tender.

5. Stir in cherry tomatoes and cook for 1-2 minutes, until they start to soften. Season with salt and pepper to taste.

6. Once the veggies are cooked, remove them from the skillet and set aside.

7. In the same skillet, add the marinated shrimp in a single layer. Cook for 2-3 minutes per side, or until they turn pink and opaque.

8. Once the shrimp are cooked, return the cooked veggies to the skillet and toss everything together to combine.

9. Serve the Cajun Shrimp and Veggie mixture over a bed of creamy veggie grits.

10. Garnish with chopped fresh parsley and grated cheese if desired.

11. Enjoy your delicious and nutritious Cajun Shrimp with Veggie Grits!

Mediterranean Salmon with Sun-Dried Tomatoes and Spinach

Ingredients:

- 4 salmon filets (about 6 ounces each), skinless
- Salt and pepper to taste
- 2 tablespoons olive oil
- 4 cloves garlic, minced
- 1/4 cup sun-dried tomatoes, chopped
- 2 cups fresh spinach leaves
- 1/4 cup Kalamata olives, pitted and sliced
- Juice of 1 lemon
- 1 teaspoon dried oregano
- 1 teaspoon dried basil
- 1/4 cup crumbled feta cheese (optional)

- Fresh parsley for garnish

Directions:

1. Preheat your oven to 400°F (200°C). Line a baking sheet with parchment paper.
2. Season the salmon filets with salt and pepper to taste on both sides.
3. Heat olive oil in a large oven-safe skillet over medium heat. Add minced garlic and sauté for 1 minute until fragrant.
4. Add chopped sun-dried tomatoes to the skillet and cook for 1-2 minutes.
5. Add fresh spinach leaves to the skillet and cook until wilted, about 2-3 minutes.
6. Stir in sliced Kalamata olives, lemon juice, dried oregano, and dried basil. Cook for another 1-2 minutes, stirring occasionally.
7. Push the spinach mixture to the sides of the skillet and place the salmon filets in the center.
8. Transfer the skillet to the preheated oven and bake for 12-15 minutes, or until the salmon is cooked through and flakes easily with a fork.
9. Once the salmon is cooked, remove the skillet from the oven.
10. Garnish the Mediterranean Salmon with crumbled feta cheese (if using) and fresh parsley.
11. Serve the salmon filets with the spinach mixture on the side.
12. Enjoy your delicious and nutritious Mediterranean Salmon with Sun-Dried Tomatoes and Spinach!

Coconut Curry Mussels with Brown Rice

Ingredients:

For the Coconut Curry Mussels:

- 2 pounds fresh mussels, cleaned and debearded

- 1 tablespoon olive oil

- 1 small onion, finely chopped

- 2 cloves garlic, minced

- 1 tablespoon curry powder

- 1 teaspoon ground turmeric

- 1 teaspoon ground cumin

- 1 teaspoon ground coriander

- 1 can (14 ounces) coconut milk

- Juice of 1 lime

- Salt and pepper to taste

- Fresh cilantro for garnish

For the Brown Rice:

- 1 cup brown rice

- 2 cups water or low-sodium chicken broth

- Salt to taste

Directions:

1. In a large pot or Dutch oven, heat olive oil over medium heat. Add chopped onion and minced garlic, and sauté until softened and fragrant, about 2-3 minutes.

2. Stir in curry powder, ground turmeric, ground cumin, and ground coriander. Cook for another minute to toast the spices.

3. Pour in the coconut milk and stir well to combine with the spices. Bring the mixture to a simmer.

4. Add cleaned and debearded mussels to the pot. Cover and cook for 5-7 minutes, or until the mussels have opened. Discard any mussels that do not open.

5. While the mussels are cooking, prepare the brown rice. In a separate saucepan, combine brown rice, water or chicken broth, and salt to taste. Bring to a boil, then reduce the heat to low, cover, and simmer for 35-40 minutes, or until the rice is tender and the liquid is absorbed.

6. Once the mussels are cooked and the rice is ready, stir in the lime juice and season the coconut curry broth with salt and pepper to taste.

7. Serve the Coconut Curry Mussels over cooked brown rice.

8. Garnish with fresh cilantro leaves.

9. Enjoy your flavorful and nutritious Coconut Curry Mussels with Brown Rice!

Pan-Seared Scallops with Lemon Butter Sauce and Quinoa

Ingredients:

For the Pan-Seared Scallops:

- 1 lb fresh scallops, side muscle removed
- Salt and pepper to taste
- 2 tablespoons olive oil

For the Lemon Butter Sauce:

- 4 tablespoons unsalted butter
- 2 cloves garlic, minced
- Zest and juice of 1 lemon
- 2 tablespoons chopped fresh parsley
- Salt and pepper to taste

For the Quinoa:

- 1 cup quinoa, rinsed
- 2 cups water or low-sodium chicken broth

- Salt to taste

- Chopped fresh parsley for garnish

Directions:

1. Start by cooking the quinoa. In a medium saucepan, combine quinoa, water or chicken broth, and salt to taste. Bring to a boil, then reduce the heat to low, cover, and simmer for 15-20 minutes, or until the quinoa is tender and the liquid is absorbed. Fluff the quinoa with a fork and set aside.

2. While the quinoa is cooking, prepare the lemon butter sauce. In a small saucepan, melt the unsalted butter over medium heat. Add minced garlic and cook for 1-2 minutes until fragrant.

3. Stir in the lemon zest, lemon juice, and chopped fresh parsley. Season with salt and pepper to taste. Keep the sauce warm over low heat while you cook the scallops.

4. Pat the scallops dry with paper towels to remove any excess moisture. Season both sides of the scallops with salt and pepper.

5. Heat olive oil in a large skillet over medium-high heat. Once the skillet is hot, add the scallops in a single layer, making sure not to overcrowd the pan. Cook for 2-3 minutes per side, or until golden brown and caramelized.

6. Once the scallops are cooked, remove them from the skillet and transfer them to a plate.

7. To serve, spoon the cooked quinoa onto plates or bowls. Arrange the pan-seared scallops on top of the quinoa.

8. Drizzle the lemon butter sauce over the scallops and quinoa.

9. Garnish with chopped fresh parsley.

10. Enjoy your delicious and nutritious Pan-Seared Scallops with Lemon Butter Sauce and Quinoa!

Baked Cod with Panko Herb Crust and Roasted Sweet Potato Fries

Ingredients:

For the Baked Cod:

- 4 cod filets (about 6 ounces each)
- Salt and pepper to taste
- 1 tablespoon olive oil

For the Panko Herb Crust:

- 1 cup panko breadcrumbs
- 2 tablespoons grated Parmesan cheese
- 1 teaspoon dried parsley
- 1 teaspoon dried thyme
- 1 teaspoon dried oregano
- 1/2 teaspoon garlic powder
- 1/4 teaspoon paprika
- Salt and pepper to taste
- 2 tablespoons melted butter or olive oil

For the Roasted Sweet Potato Fries:

- 2 large sweet potatoes, peeled and cut into fries
- 2 tablespoons olive oil
- 1 teaspoon garlic powder
- 1 teaspoon paprika
- Salt and pepper to taste

Directions:

1. Preheat your oven to 400°F (200°C). Line a baking sheet with parchment paper.

2. Pat the cod filets dry with paper towels and season them with salt and pepper to taste.

3. Place the cod filets on the prepared baking sheet and drizzle them with olive oil.

4. In a small bowl, mix together panko breadcrumbs, grated Parmesan cheese, dried parsley, dried thyme, dried oregano, garlic powder, paprika, salt, and pepper.

5. Brush each cod filet with melted butter or olive oil, then press the panko herb crust mixture onto the top of each filet.

6. Arrange the sweet potato fries on the same baking sheet. Drizzle them with olive oil and sprinkle with garlic powder, paprika, salt, and pepper.

7. Transfer the baking sheet to the preheated oven and bake for 15-20 minutes, or until the cod is cooked through and the crust is golden brown, and the sweet potato fries are tender and crispy, flipping the fries halfway through.

8. Once the cod and sweet potato fries are done baking, remove them from the oven.

9. Serve the Baked Cod with Panko Herb Crust alongside the Roasted Sweet Potato Fries.

10. Enjoy your delicious and nutritious meal!

Tuna Noodle Casserole with Whole-Wheat Noodles and Light Cream Sauce

Ingredients:

- 8 ounces whole-wheat egg noodles
- 2 tablespoons olive oil
- 1 onion, diced
- 2 cloves garlic, minced
- 2 cups sliced mushrooms
- 2 cups frozen peas, thawed
- 2 cans (5 ounces each) tuna in water, drained
- 2 tablespoons all-purpose flour
- 1 1/2 cups low-fat milk
- 1/2 cup low-sodium chicken or vegetable broth
- 1/2 teaspoon dried thyme
- 1/2 teaspoon dried parsley
- Salt and pepper to taste
- 1/2 cup grated Parmesan cheese
- 1/2 cup whole-wheat breadcrumbs

Directions:

1. Preheat your oven to 375°F (190°C). Grease a 9x13-inch baking dish with cooking spray.
2. Cook the whole-wheat egg noodles according to the package instructions until al dente. Drain and set aside.
3. In a large skillet, heat olive oil over medium heat. Add diced onion and minced garlic, and cook until softened, about 3-4 minutes.

4. Add sliced mushrooms to the skillet and cook until they release their moisture and become tender, about 5 minutes.

5. Stir in the thawed peas and drained tuna, and cook for another 2-3 minutes to heat through.

6. Sprinkle the flour over the mixture in the skillet and stir to coat everything evenly.

7. Slowly pour in the low-fat milk and chicken or vegetable broth, stirring constantly to prevent lumps from forming.

8. Add dried thyme, dried parsley, salt, and pepper to taste. Cook, stirring occasionally, until the sauce thickens, about 5-7 minutes.

9. Add the cooked whole-wheat egg noodles to the skillet and toss everything together until well combined.

10. Transfer the mixture to the prepared baking dish and spread it out evenly.

11. In a small bowl, combine grated Parmesan cheese and whole-wheat breadcrumbs. Sprinkle this mixture over the top of the casserole.

12. Bake in the preheated oven for 20-25 minutes, or until the top is golden brown and the casserole is bubbling around the edges.

13. Remove from the oven and let it cool slightly before serving.

14. Enjoy your healthier Tuna Noodle Casserole with Whole-Wheat Noodles and Light Cream Sauce!

Spicy Shrimp Fajitas with Whole-Wheat Tortillas and Grilled Vegetables

Ingredients:

For the Spicy Shrimp:

- 1 lb large shrimp, peeled and deveined

- 2 tablespoons olive oil
- 2 cloves garlic, minced
- 1 teaspoon chili powder
- 1/2 teaspoon cumin
- 1/2 teaspoon paprika
- 1/4 teaspoon cayenne pepper (adjust to taste)
- Salt and pepper to taste
- Juice of 1 lime

For the Grilled Vegetables:

- 1 red bell pepper, sliced
- 1 green bell pepper, sliced
- 1 yellow bell pepper, sliced
- 1 onion, sliced
- 2 tablespoons olive oil
- Salt and pepper to taste

For Serving:

- Whole-wheat tortillas
- Sliced avocado
- Fresh cilantro leaves
- Lime wedges

Directions:

1. Preheat your grill or grill pan over medium-high heat.
2. In a large bowl, combine peeled and deveined shrimp with olive oil, minced garlic, chili powder, cumin, paprika, cayenne pepper, salt, pepper, and lime juice. Toss until the shrimp are evenly coated in the marinade.

3. Thread the marinated shrimp on skewers if using, or simply place them directly on the grill. Cook for 2-3 minutes per side, or until the shrimp are pink and opaque. Remove from the grill and set aside.

4. While the shrimp are cooking, prepare the grilled vegetables. In a large bowl, toss sliced bell peppers and onion with olive oil, salt, and pepper until evenly coated.

5. Place the seasoned vegetables on the grill and cook for 4-5 minutes per side, or until they are tender and slightly charred. Remove from the grill and set aside.

6. Warm the whole-wheat tortillas on the grill for about 30 seconds per side, or until they are heated through and slightly charred.

7. To assemble the fajitas, place a few grilled shrimp and some grilled vegetables in the center of each tortilla. Top with sliced avocado and fresh cilantro leaves.

8. Serve the Spicy Shrimp Fajitas with lime wedges on the side for squeezing over the top.

9. Enjoy your delicious and nutritious meal!

Poached Salmon with Creamy Dill Sauce and Roasted Brussels Sprouts

Ingredients:

For the Poached Salmon:

- 4 salmon filets (about 6 ounces each), skin removed
- 4 cups water or vegetable broth
- 1 lemon, sliced
- 2 bay leaves
- Salt and pepper to taste

For the Creamy Dill Sauce:

- 1/2 cup plain Greek yogurt
- 2 tablespoons mayonnaise
- 1 tablespoon chopped fresh dill
- 1 tablespoon lemon juice
- 1 clove garlic, minced
- Salt and pepper to taste

For the Roasted Brussels Sprouts:

- 1 lb Brussels sprouts, trimmed and halved
- 2 tablespoons olive oil
- Salt and pepper to taste

Directions:

1. Preheat your oven to 400°F (200°C).

2. In a large skillet or shallow pan, bring water or vegetable broth to a gentle simmer over medium heat. Add lemon slices and bay leaves to the simmering liquid.

3. Season the salmon filets with salt and pepper on both sides. Carefully add the seasoned salmon filets to the simmering liquid, ensuring they are fully submerged.

4. Poach the salmon for 8-10 minutes, or until the fish is cooked through and flakes easily with a fork. Remove the salmon from the poaching liquid and set aside.

5. While the salmon is poaching, prepare the creamy dill sauce. In a small bowl, combine Greek yogurt, mayonnaise, chopped fresh dill, lemon juice, minced garlic, salt, and pepper. Stir until well combined. Adjust the seasoning to taste.

6. In a large mixing bowl, toss halved Brussels sprouts with olive oil, salt, and pepper until evenly coated. Spread the Brussels sprouts out in a single layer on a baking sheet lined with parchment paper.

7. Roast the Brussels sprouts in the preheated oven for 20-25 minutes, or until they are tender and caramelized, stirring halfway through cooking.

8. Once the salmon is poached and the Brussels sprouts are roasted, divide the salmon filets and Brussels sprouts among serving plates.

9. Drizzle the creamy dill sauce over the poached salmon filets.

10. Serve immediately and enjoy your delicious and nutritious Poached Salmon with Creamy Dill Sauce and Roasted Brussels Sprouts!

Grilled Swordfish with Mango Salsa and Black Beans

Ingredients:

For the Grilled Swordfish:

- 4 swordfish steaks (about 6 ounces each)
- 2 tablespoons olive oil
- 2 cloves garlic, minced
- 1 teaspoon smoked paprika
- 1 teaspoon ground cumin
- Salt and pepper to taste
- Lime wedges for serving

For the Mango Salsa:

- 1 ripe mango, peeled, pitted, and diced
- 1/2 red bell pepper, diced
- 1/4 red onion, finely chopped
- 1 jalapeño pepper, seeded and minced

- Juice of 1 lime

- 2 tablespoons chopped fresh cilantro

- Salt and pepper to taste

For the Black Beans:

- 1 can (15 ounces) black beans, drained and rinsed

- 2 cloves garlic, minced

- 1/2 teaspoon ground cumin

- 1/2 teaspoon chili powder

- Salt and pepper to taste

- Chopped fresh cilantro for garnish

Directions:

1. Preheat your grill to medium-high heat.

2. In a small bowl, mix together olive oil, minced garlic, smoked paprika, ground cumin, salt, and pepper to make a marinade for the swordfish.

3. Pat the swordfish steaks dry with paper towels. Brush both sides of the swordfish steaks with the marinade.

4. In another bowl, combine diced mango, diced red bell pepper, finely chopped red onion, minced jalapeño pepper, lime juice, chopped fresh cilantro, salt, and pepper to make the mango salsa. Stir well to combine and set aside.

5. In a small saucepan, heat a tablespoon of olive oil over medium heat. Add minced garlic and cook for about 30 seconds, until fragrant.

6. Add drained and rinsed black beans to the saucepan. Stir in ground cumin, chili powder, salt, and pepper. Cook for 3-4 minutes, stirring occasionally, until heated through.

7. Place the marinated swordfish steaks on the preheated grill. Grill for 4-5 minutes per side, or until the fish is cooked through and easily flakes with a fork.

8. While the swordfish is grilling, gently warm the black beans on the stovetop over low heat, stirring occasionally.

9. Once the swordfish is done, remove it from the grill and let it rest for a few minutes.

10. To serve, spoon some black beans onto each plate. Top with grilled swordfish steaks and a generous portion of mango salsa.

11. Garnish with chopped fresh cilantro and serve with lime wedges on the side.

12. Enjoy your delicious and nutritious Grilled Swordfish with Mango Salsa and Black Beans!

Salmon Burgers with Avocado Mayo and Whole-Wheat Buns

Ingredients:

For the Salmon Burgers:
- 1 lb fresh salmon filet, skin removed
- 1/4 cup whole-wheat breadcrumbs
- 1/4 cup finely chopped red onion
- 2 tablespoons chopped fresh parsley
- 1 clove garlic, minced
- 1 teaspoon Dijon mustard
- 1 egg, beaten
- Salt and pepper to taste
- Olive oil for cooking

For the Avocado Mayo:

- 1 ripe avocado, peeled and pitted
- 2 tablespoons Greek yogurt
- 1 tablespoon lemon juice
- Salt and pepper to taste

For Serving:

- Whole-wheat burger buns
- Lettuce leaves
- Sliced tomatoes
- Sliced red onion

Directions:

1. Begin by making the avocado mayo. In a small bowl, mash the ripe avocado with a fork until smooth. Stir in Greek yogurt, lemon juice, salt, and pepper until well combined. Set aside.

2. Cut the fresh salmon filet into small chunks. Place the salmon chunks in a food processor and pulse until finely chopped, but not pureed. Transfer the chopped salmon to a large mixing bowl.

3. To the bowl with the chopped salmon, add whole-wheat breadcrumbs, finely chopped red onion, chopped fresh parsley, minced garlic, Dijon mustard, beaten egg, salt, and pepper. Mix until all ingredients are well combined.

4. Divide the salmon mixture into four equal portions and shape each portion into a patty.

5. Heat olive oil in a large skillet over medium heat. Once the skillet is hot, add the salmon patties and cook for 4-5 minutes on each side, or until golden brown and cooked through.

6. While the salmon burgers are cooking, toast the whole-wheat burger buns until lightly golden.

7. To assemble the burgers, spread a generous amount of avocado mayo on the bottom half of each toasted bun. Top with a lettuce leaf, a salmon patty, sliced tomatoes, and sliced red onion. Place the top half of the bun on top.

8. Serve the Salmon Burgers with Avocado Mayo immediately, and enjoy!

Shrimp and Vegetable Stir-Fry with Brown Rice Noodles

Ingredients:

For the Stir-Fry Sauce:

- 1/4 cup low-sodium soy sauce
- 2 tablespoons oyster sauce
- 1 tablespoon rice vinegar
- 1 tablespoon honey or maple syrup
- 1 teaspoon sesame oil
- 2 cloves garlic, minced
- 1 teaspoon grated ginger
- 1 tablespoon cornstarch
- 1/4 cup water

For the Stir-Fry:

- 8 ounces brown rice noodles
- 1 tablespoon olive oil or sesame oil
- 1 lb large shrimp, peeled and deveined
- 2 cups mixed vegetables (such as bell peppers, broccoli, snap peas, carrots, and mushrooms), sliced

- Salt and pepper to taste

- Sesame seeds and chopped green onions for garnish (optional)

Directions:

1. In a small bowl, whisk together all the ingredients for the stir-fry sauce: low-sodium soy sauce, oyster sauce, rice vinegar, honey or maple syrup, sesame oil, minced garlic, grated ginger, cornstarch, and water. Set aside.

2. Cook the brown rice noodles according to the package instructions until al dente. Drain and set aside.

3. Heat olive oil or sesame oil in a large skillet or wok over medium-high heat. Add the shrimp and cook for 2-3 minutes, or until they turn pink and opaque. Remove the shrimp from the skillet and set aside.

4. In the same skillet, add more oil if needed, then add the mixed vegetables. Stir-fry for 3-4 minutes, or until the vegetables are tender-crisp.

5. Return the cooked shrimp to the skillet with the vegetables.

6. Pour the prepared stir-fry sauce over the shrimp and vegetables. Cook, stirring constantly, for 1-2 minutes, or until the sauce thickens and coats the shrimp and vegetables evenly.

7. Add the cooked brown rice noodles to the skillet and toss everything together until well combined.

8. Season with salt and pepper to taste.

9. Garnish with sesame seeds and chopped green onions, if desired.

10. Serve the Shrimp and Vegetable Stir-Fry with Brown Rice Noodles immediately and enjoy!

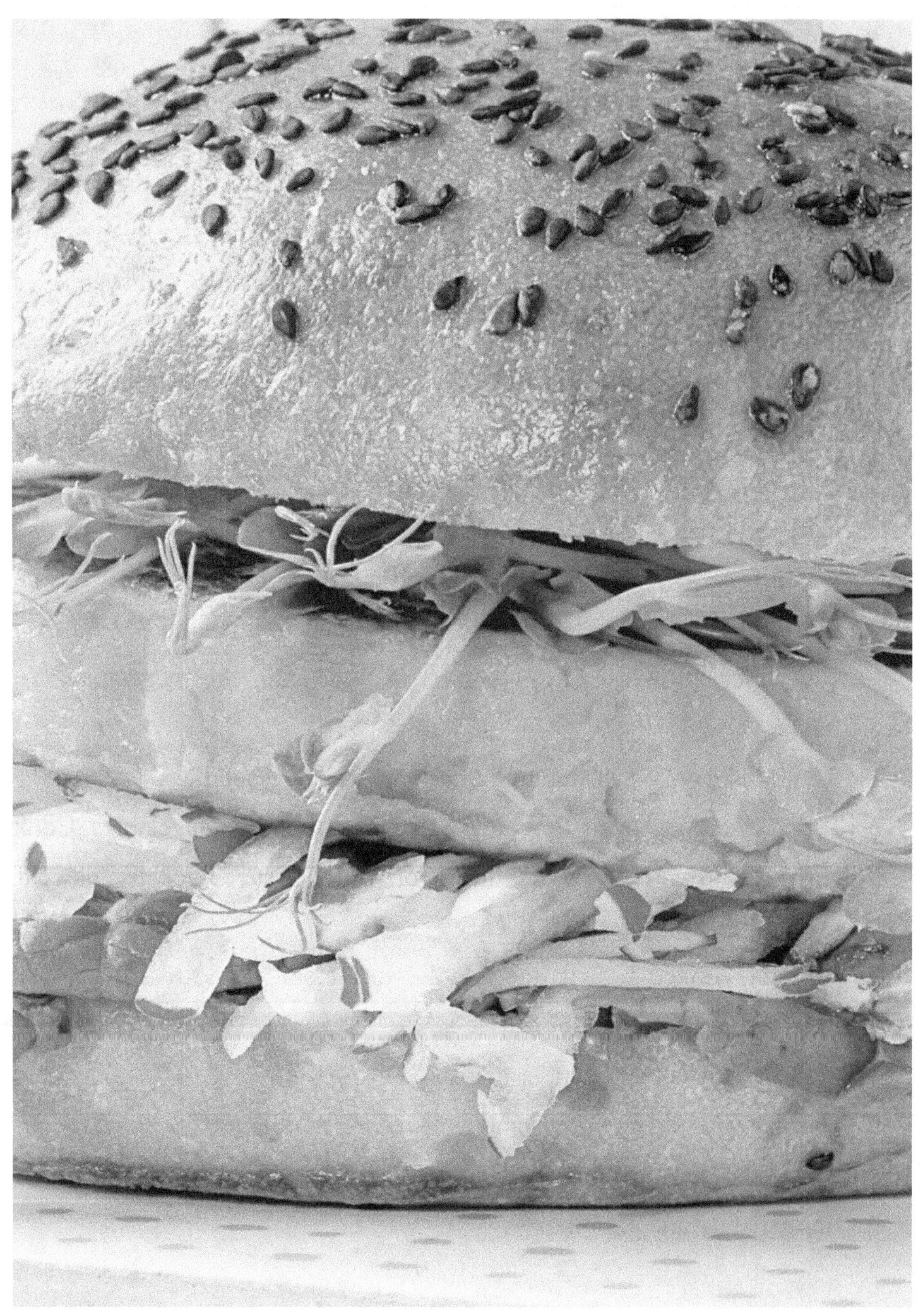

Chapter 9: Vegetarian Recipes

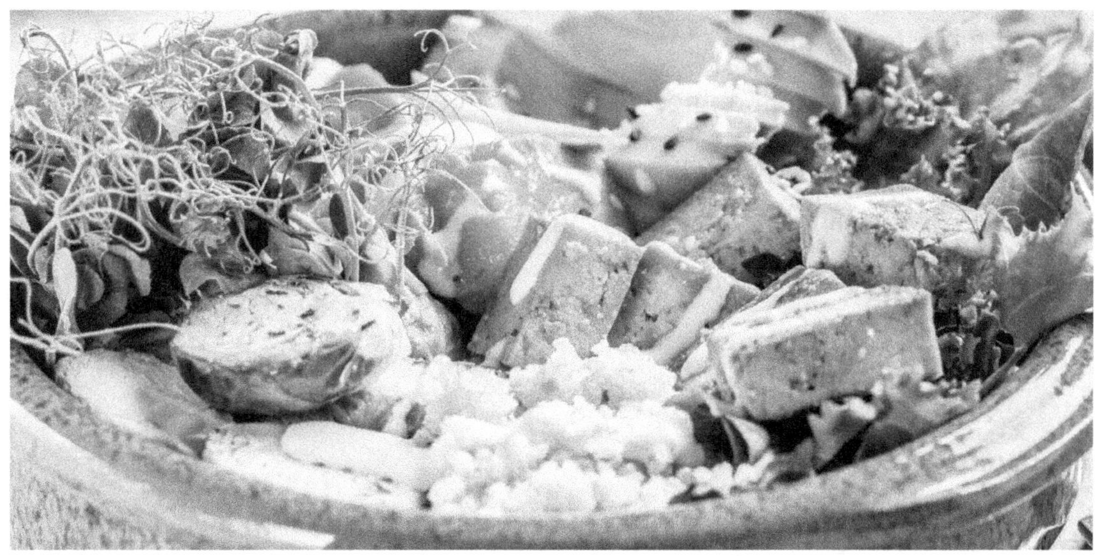

Veggie-Packed Buddha Bowl with Quinoa and Tahini Dressing

Ingredients:

For the Buddha Bowl:

- 1 cup cooked quinoa
- 1 cup mixed greens (such as spinach, kale, or arugula)
- 1/2 cup cherry tomatoes, halved
- 1/2 cup cucumber, diced
- 1/2 cup bell peppers, sliced
- 1/2 cup shredded carrots
- 1/4 cup red cabbage, shredded
- 1/4 cup cooked chickpeas
- 1/4 cup sliced avocado
- 2 tablespoons pumpkin seeds (pepitas), toasted

- Salt and pepper to taste

For the Tahini Dressing:

- 2 tablespoons tahini
- 2 tablespoons lemon juice
- 1 tablespoon olive oil
- 1 teaspoon honey or maple syrup (optional)
- 1 clove garlic, minced
- 2-3 tablespoons water (adjust for desired consistency)
- Salt and pepper to taste

Directions:

1. Prepare the quinoa according to package instructions and set aside.
2. In a small bowl, whisk together the tahini, lemon juice, olive oil, honey or maple syrup (if using), minced garlic, salt, and pepper. Gradually add water, a tablespoon at a time, until you reach your desired dressing consistency. Set aside.
3. Assemble the Buddha bowls by dividing the cooked quinoa, mixed greens, cherry tomatoes, cucumber, bell peppers, shredded carrots, red cabbage, cooked chickpeas, sliced avocado, and toasted pumpkin seeds evenly among serving bowls.
4. Drizzle each Buddha bowl with the tahini dressing.
5. Season with salt and pepper to taste.
6. Serve immediately and enjoy your Veggie-Packed Buddha Bowl with Quinoa and Tahini Dressing!

Stuffed Portobello Mushrooms with Goat Cheese and Spinach

Ingredients:

- 4 large portobello mushrooms, stems removed
- 2 cups fresh spinach, chopped
- 1 tablespoon olive oil
- 2 cloves garlic, minced
- 4 ounces goat cheese, crumbled
- 2 tablespoons grated Parmesan cheese
- Salt and pepper to taste
- Fresh parsley, chopped (for garnish)

Directions:

1. Preheat your oven to 375°F (190°C). Line a baking sheet with parchment paper or lightly grease it with olive oil.
2. Clean the portobello mushrooms by gently wiping them with a damp paper towel. Remove the stems and carefully scoop out the gills using a spoon. Place the mushrooms on the prepared baking sheet, gill-side up.
3. In a skillet, heat olive oil over medium heat. Add minced garlic and sauté for 1-2 minutes, until fragrant.
4. Add chopped spinach to the skillet and cook until wilted, about 2-3 minutes. Season with salt and pepper to taste.
5. Remove the skillet from heat and let the spinach mixture cool slightly.
6. Once cooled, stir in crumbled goat cheese until well combined.
7. Divide the spinach and goat cheese mixture evenly among the portobello mushrooms, filling each mushroom cap.
8. Sprinkle grated Parmesan cheese over the stuffed mushrooms.

9. Bake in the preheated oven for 15-20 minutes, or until the mushrooms are tender and the cheese is melted and bubbly.

10. Remove from the oven and let the stuffed mushrooms cool for a few minutes before serving.

11. Garnish with chopped fresh parsley before serving, if desired.

12. Serve your Stuffed Portobello Mushrooms with Goat Cheese and Spinach as a delicious and satisfying meal.

Black Bean Burgers with Sweet Potato Buns

Ingredients:

For the Black Bean Burgers:

- 2 cans (15 ounces each) black beans, drained and rinsed
- 1 cup cooked quinoa
- 1/2 cup finely chopped onion
- 1/2 cup finely chopped bell pepper (any color)
- 2 cloves garlic, minced
- 1 teaspoon ground cumin
- 1 teaspoon chili powder
- 1/2 teaspoon smoked paprika
- Salt and pepper to taste
- 1 tablespoon olive oil (for cooking)

For the Sweet Potato Buns:

- 2 large sweet potatoes, peeled and sliced into 1/2-inch rounds
- Olive oil, for brushing
- Salt and pepper to taste

For Serving:

- Burger toppings of your choice (lettuce, tomato, avocado, onion, etc.)

Directions:

1. Preheat your oven to 400°F (200°C).

2. Place the sliced sweet potatoes on a baking sheet lined with parchment paper. Brush both sides of the sweet potato rounds with olive oil and season with salt and pepper.

3. Bake the sweet potato rounds in the preheated oven for 20-25 minutes, flipping halfway through, or until tender and lightly browned.

4. While the sweet potatoes are baking, prepare the black bean burgers. In a large mixing bowl, mash the black beans with a fork or potato masher until mostly smooth but with some chunks remaining.

5. Add cooked quinoa, chopped onion, chopped bell pepper, minced garlic, ground cumin, chili powder, smoked paprika, salt, and pepper to the mashed black beans. Mix until well combined.

6. Divide the black bean mixture into four equal portions and shape each portion into a burger patty.

7. Heat olive oil in a large skillet over medium heat. Once hot, add the black bean burgers to the skillet and cook for 4-5 minutes on each side, or until golden brown and heated through.

8. Once the sweet potato rounds are done baking, assemble your burgers by placing a black bean burger patty on top of a sweet potato round. Add your desired toppings and another sweet potato round on top to create a burger "sandwich."

9. Serve your Black Bean Burgers with Sweet Potato Buns immediately and enjoy!

Lentil Soup with Whole-Wheat Bread and a dollop of Greek Yogurt

Ingredients:

For the Lentil Soup:

- 1 cup dried green or brown lentils, rinsed and drained
- 1 tablespoon olive oil
- 1 onion, diced
- 2 carrots, diced
- 2 celery stalks, diced
- 3 cloves garlic, minced
- 1 teaspoon ground cumin
- 1 teaspoon ground turmeric
- 1/2 teaspoon ground coriander
- 6 cups vegetable broth
- 1 bay leaf
- Salt and pepper to taste
- Fresh parsley or cilantro, chopped (for garnish)

For Serving:

- Whole-wheat bread slices
- Greek yogurt

Directions:

1. In a large pot, heat olive oil over medium heat. Add diced onion, carrots, and celery, and cook until softened, about 5-7 minutes.
2. Add minced garlic, ground cumin, ground turmeric, and ground coriander to the pot. Cook for another minute, stirring constantly, until fragrant.

3. Add rinsed and drained lentils to the pot, along with vegetable broth and bay leaf. Stir to combine.

4. Bring the soup to a boil, then reduce the heat to low and simmer, partially covered, for about 20-25 minutes, or until the lentils are tender.

5. Season the soup with salt and pepper to taste. Adjust the seasoning if needed.

6. Once the lentils are cooked, remove the bay leaf from the soup.

7. To serve, ladle the hot lentil soup into bowls. Garnish each bowl with chopped fresh parsley or cilantro.

8. Serve the Lentil Soup with slices of whole-wheat bread on the side.

9. Add a dollop of Greek yogurt on top of each bowl of soup before serving.

10. Enjoy your delicious and nutritious Lentil Soup with Whole-Wheat Bread and Greek Yogurt!

Vegetable Quesadillas with Whole-Wheat Tortillas and Low-Fat Cheese

Ingredients:

- 4 whole-wheat tortillas
- 1 cup low-fat shredded cheese (such as cheddar or mozzarella)
- 1 red bell pepper, thinly sliced
- 1 green bell pepper, thinly sliced
- 1 small zucchini, thinly sliced
- 1 small yellow squash, thinly sliced
- 1 small red onion, thinly sliced
- 1 tablespoon olive oil
- 1 teaspoon ground cumin

- 1 teaspoon chili powder

- Salt and pepper to taste

- Salsa, guacamole, or Greek yogurt for serving (optional)

Directions:

1. Heat olive oil in a large skillet over medium heat. Add sliced red bell pepper, green bell pepper, zucchini, yellow squash, and red onion to the skillet.

2. Season the vegetables with ground cumin, chili powder, salt, and pepper. Cook, stirring occasionally, for 5-7 minutes, or until the vegetables are tender-crisp. Remove from heat and set aside.

3. Preheat a large non-stick skillet or griddle over medium heat.

4. Place one whole-wheat tortilla on the preheated skillet. Sprinkle 1/4 cup of low-fat shredded cheese evenly over the tortilla.

5. Spoon a portion of the cooked vegetable mixture evenly over one half of the tortilla.

6. Fold the other half of the tortilla over the filling to create a half-moon shape.

7. Cook the quesadilla for 2-3 minutes on each side, or until the tortilla is golden brown and the cheese is melted.

8. Remove the cooked quesadilla from the skillet and repeat the process with the remaining tortillas, cheese, and vegetable mixture.

9. Once all the quesadillas are cooked, cut each quesadilla into wedges using a sharp knife or pizza cutter.

10. Serve the Vegetable Quesadillas with Whole-Wheat Tortillas and Low-Fat Cheese with salsa, guacamole, or Greek yogurt on the side for dipping, if desired.

11. Enjoy your delicious and nutritious Vegetable Quesadillas!

Vegetable Frittata with Goat Cheese and Herbs

Ingredients:

- 8 large eggs
- 1/4 cup milk or unsweetened almond milk
- Salt and pepper to taste
- 1 tablespoon olive oil
- 1 small onion, diced
- 1 bell pepper, diced
- 1 cup sliced mushrooms
- 2 cups baby spinach
- 2 ounces goat cheese, crumbled
- 2 tablespoons chopped fresh herbs (such as parsley, thyme, or basil)

Directions:

1. Preheat your oven to 350°F (175°C).
2. In a large mixing bowl, whisk together the eggs, milk, salt, and pepper until well combined. Set aside.
3. Heat olive oil in a large oven-safe skillet over medium heat. Add diced onion and bell pepper to the skillet and cook for 3-4 minutes, or until softened.
4. Add sliced mushrooms to the skillet and cook for another 2-3 minutes, or until they release their moisture and start to brown.
5. Add baby spinach to the skillet and cook for 1-2 minutes, or until wilted.
6. Pour the egg mixture over the cooked vegetables in the skillet. Use a spatula to gently stir the mixture, distributing the vegetables evenly.
7. Crumble goat cheese evenly over the top of the frittata mixture.
8. Sprinkle chopped fresh herbs over the top of the frittata.

9. Transfer the skillet to the preheated oven and bake for 15-20 minutes, or until the frittata is set in the center and the edges are lightly golden brown.

10. Once done, remove the skillet from the oven and let the frittata cool for a few minutes before slicing.

11. Slice the Vegetable Frittata with Goat Cheese and Herbs into wedges and serve warm.

12. Enjoy your delicious and nutritious Vegetable Frittata!

Creamy Tomato Pasta with Chickpeas and Spinach

Ingredients:

- 8 ounces whole wheat pasta
- 1 tablespoon olive oil
- 3 cloves garlic, minced
- 1 can (15 ounces) chickpeas, drained and rinsed
- 1 can (14.5 ounces) diced tomatoes, with juices
- 1/2 cup vegetable broth
- 1 teaspoon dried basil
- 1 teaspoon dried oregano
- 1/2 teaspoon red pepper flakes (optional)
- Salt and pepper to taste
- 2 cups baby spinach
- 1/4 cup plain Greek yogurt (optional, for extra creaminess)
- Grated Parmesan cheese for serving (optional)
- Fresh basil leaves for garnish (optional)

Directions:

1. Cook the whole wheat pasta according to the package instructions until al dente. Drain and set aside.

2. In a large skillet, heat olive oil over medium heat. Add minced garlic and cook for about 1 minute, or until fragrant.

3. Add chickpeas to the skillet and cook for 3-4 minutes, stirring occasionally, until lightly browned.

4. Stir in diced tomatoes (with juices), vegetable broth, dried basil, dried oregano, red pepper flakes (if using), salt, and pepper. Bring the mixture to a simmer and cook for 5-7 minutes, allowing the flavors to meld together and the sauce to thicken slightly.

5. Add baby spinach to the skillet and cook for 1-2 minutes, or until wilted.

6. If desired, stir in plain Greek yogurt for extra creaminess.

7. Add the cooked whole wheat pasta to the skillet and toss everything together until the pasta is well coated with the creamy tomato sauce.

8. Taste and adjust seasoning as needed, adding more salt, pepper, or herbs if desired.

9. Serve the Creamy Tomato Pasta with Chickpeas and Spinach hot, garnished with grated Parmesan cheese and fresh basil leaves if desired.

10. Enjoy your delicious and nutritious Creamy Tomato Pasta!

Tofu Scramble with Whole-Wheat Toast and Avocado

Ingredients:

For the Tofu Scramble:

*   1 tablespoon olive oil

- 1 block (14 ounces) firm tofu, drained and pressed
- 1/2 onion, diced
- 1 bell pepper, diced
- 2 cloves garlic, minced
- 1 teaspoon ground turmeric
- 1/2 teaspoon ground cumin
- 1/2 teaspoon smoked paprika
- Salt and pepper to taste
- 2 cups baby spinach
- 1 tablespoon nutritional yeast (optional, for added flavor)
- Fresh parsley or cilantro, chopped (for garnish)

For Serving:

- Whole-wheat toast slices
- Avocado slices

Directions:

1. Heat olive oil in a large skillet over medium heat.
2. Crumble the pressed tofu into the skillet using your hands or a fork, resembling scrambled eggs.
3. Add diced onion and bell pepper to the skillet. Cook for 5-7 minutes, or until the vegetables are softened.
4. Stir in minced garlic, ground turmeric, ground cumin, smoked paprika, salt, and pepper. Cook for another minute, stirring constantly, until the spices are fragrant.
5. Add baby spinach to the skillet and cook for 1-2 minutes, or until wilted.
6. If using, sprinkle nutritional yeast over the tofu scramble and stir to combine.

7. Taste and adjust seasoning as needed, adding more salt and pepper if desired.

8. Remove the skillet from heat and garnish the tofu scramble with chopped fresh parsley or cilantro.

9. Serve the Tofu Scramble with Whole-Wheat Toast and Avocado slices on the side.

10. Enjoy your delicious and nutritious meal!

Roasted Eggplant with Lentil Bolognese

Ingredients:

For the Roasted Eggplant:

- 2 large eggplants, sliced lengthwise
- 2 tablespoons olive oil
- Salt and pepper to taste

For the Lentil Bolognese:

- 1 cup dried brown lentils, rinsed and drained
- 2 tablespoons olive oil
- 1 onion, diced
- 2 carrots, diced
- 2 celery stalks, diced
- 3 cloves garlic, minced
- 1 can (14.5 ounces) diced tomatoes
- 1 can (6 ounces) tomato paste
- 1 teaspoon dried oregano
- 1 teaspoon dried basil
- Salt and pepper to taste
- Fresh basil leaves for garnish (optional)

- Grated Parmesan cheese for serving (optional)

Directions:

1. Preheat your oven to 400°F (200°C).

2. Place the sliced eggplants on a baking sheet lined with parchment paper. Brush both sides of the eggplant slices with olive oil and season with salt and pepper.

3. Roast the eggplant slices in the preheated oven for 20-25 minutes, flipping halfway through, or until tender and lightly browned. Remove from the oven and set aside.

4. In the meantime, cook the brown lentils according to the package instructions until tender. Drain and set aside.

5. Heat olive oil in a large skillet over medium heat. Add diced onion, carrots, and celery to the skillet and cook until softened, about 5-7 minutes.

6. Add minced garlic to the skillet and cook for another minute, or until fragrant.

7. Stir in diced tomatoes, tomato paste, dried oregano, dried basil, cooked brown lentils, salt, and pepper. Bring the mixture to a simmer and cook for 10-15 minutes, stirring occasionally, to allow the flavors to meld together and the sauce to thicken.

8. Taste and adjust seasoning as needed, adding more salt and pepper if desired.

9. To serve, place roasted eggplant slices on plates and spoon the lentil bolognese over the top.

10. Garnish with fresh basil leaves and grated Parmesan cheese if desired.

11. Enjoy your delicious and nutritious Roasted Eggplant with Lentil Bolognese!

Chickpea Curry with Brown Rice

Ingredients:

For the Chickpea Curry:

- 2 tablespoons olive oil
- 1 onion, diced
- 3 cloves garlic, minced
- 1 tablespoon fresh ginger, grated
- 2 teaspoons curry powder
- 1 teaspoon ground cumin
- 1 teaspoon ground coriander
- 1/2 teaspoon turmeric
- 1/4 teaspoon cayenne pepper (optional, for extra heat)
- 1 can (15 ounces) chickpeas, drained and rinsed
- 1 can (14.5 ounces) diced tomatoes
- 1 can (13.5 ounces) coconut milk
- Salt and pepper to taste
- Fresh cilantro, chopped (for garnish)

For the Brown Rice:

- 1 cup brown rice
- 2 cups water or vegetable broth
- Salt to taste

Directions:

1. Rinse the brown rice under cold water until the water runs clear. In a medium saucepan, combine the brown rice, water or vegetable broth, and a pinch of salt.

2. Bring to a boil, then reduce the heat to low, cover, and simmer for 40-45 minutes, or until the rice is tender and all the liquid is absorbed. Remove from heat and let it sit, covered, for 5 minutes. Fluff the rice with a fork before serving.

3. While the rice is cooking, heat olive oil in a large skillet over medium heat. Add diced onion and cook until softened, about 5 minutes.

4. Add minced garlic and grated ginger to the skillet and cook for another minute, until fragrant.

5. Stir in curry powder, ground cumin, ground coriander, turmeric, and cayenne pepper (if using). Cook for another minute to toast the spices.

6. Add drained and rinsed chickpeas, diced tomatoes (with juices), and coconut milk to the skillet. Stir to combine.

7. Bring the mixture to a simmer, then reduce the heat to low and let it simmer for 15-20 minutes, stirring occasionally, until the flavors are well combined and the sauce has thickened slightly.

8. Taste the chickpea curry and adjust seasoning with salt and pepper as needed.

9. Once the chickpea curry is done, serve it hot over cooked brown rice.

10. Garnish with fresh chopped cilantro before serving.

11. Enjoy your delicious and nutritious Chickpea Curry with Brown Rice!

Vegetable Stir-Fry with Tofu and Brown Rice Noodles

Ingredients:

For the Stir-Fry Sauce:

- 1/4 cup low-sodium soy sauce
- 2 tablespoons rice vinegar

- 1 tablespoon sesame oil
- 1 tablespoon honey or maple syrup
- 2 cloves garlic, minced
- 1 teaspoon grated ginger
- 1 tablespoon cornstarch
- 1/4 cup water

For the Stir-Fry:

- 8 ounces brown rice noodles
- 1 tablespoon olive oil
- 1 block (14 ounces) firm tofu, drained and pressed, cut into cubes
- 1 red bell pepper, thinly sliced
- 1 yellow bell pepper, thinly sliced
- 1 medium carrot, julienned
- 1 cup broccoli florets
- 1 cup snap peas, trimmed
- 2 green onions, chopped
- Sesame seeds and chopped cilantro for garnish (optional)

Directions:

1. In a small bowl, whisk together all the ingredients for the stir-fry sauce: soy sauce, rice vinegar, sesame oil, honey or maple syrup, minced garlic, grated ginger, cornstarch, and water. Set aside.

2. Cook the brown rice noodles according to the package instructions until al dente. Drain and rinse under cold water to stop the cooking process. Set aside.

3. Heat olive oil in a large skillet or wok over medium-high heat. Add the cubed tofu and cook until golden brown on all sides, about 5-7 minutes. Remove the tofu from the skillet and set aside.

4. In the same skillet, add a bit more oil if needed. Add the sliced red and yellow bell peppers, julienned carrot, broccoli florets, and snap peas. Stir-fry for 3-4 minutes, or until the vegetables are tender-crisp.

5. Return the cooked tofu to the skillet with the vegetables.

6. Pour the prepared stir-fry sauce over the tofu and vegetables in the skillet. Cook for another 2-3 minutes, stirring constantly, until the sauce has thickened and coats the tofu and vegetables evenly.

7. Add the cooked brown rice noodles to the skillet and toss everything together until well combined.

8. Remove the skillet from heat and garnish the Vegetable Stir-Fry with Tofu and Brown Rice Noodles with chopped green onions, sesame seeds, and chopped cilantro (if using).

9. Serve hot and enjoy your delicious and nutritious meal!

Roasted Butternut Squash Salad with Quinoa, Cranberries, and Goat Cheese

Ingredients:

For the Roasted Butternut Squash:

- 1 small butternut squash, peeled, seeded, and diced into cubes
- 2 tablespoons olive oil
- 1 tablespoon maple syrup
- Salt and pepper to taste

For the Salad:

- 1 cup quinoa, rinsed
- 2 cups water or vegetable broth
- 1/2 cup dried cranberries
- 1/4 cup chopped pecans or walnuts

- 2 ounces goat cheese, crumbled
- Fresh parsley or cilantro, chopped (for garnish)

For the Dressing:

- 3 tablespoons olive oil
- 2 tablespoons apple cider vinegar
- 1 tablespoon maple syrup
- 1 teaspoon Dijon mustard
- Salt and pepper to taste

Directions:

1. Preheat your oven to 400°F (200°C).
2. In a mixing bowl, combine the diced butternut squash with olive oil, maple syrup, salt, and pepper. Toss until the squash is evenly coated.
3. Spread the seasoned butternut squash cubes in a single layer on a baking sheet lined with parchment paper. Roast in the preheated oven for 25-30 minutes, or until tender and caramelized, flipping halfway through. Remove from the oven and let it cool slightly.
4. In the meantime, cook the quinoa. In a medium saucepan, combine the rinsed quinoa and water or vegetable broth. Bring to a boil, then reduce the heat to low, cover, and simmer for 15-20 minutes, or until the quinoa is fluffy and the liquid is absorbed. Remove from heat and let it sit, covered, for 5 minutes. Fluff the quinoa with a fork and let it cool slightly.
5. In a small bowl, whisk together the ingredients for the dressing: olive oil, apple cider vinegar, maple syrup, Dijon mustard, salt, and pepper.
6. In a large mixing bowl, combine the cooked quinoa, roasted butternut squash cubes, dried cranberries, chopped pecans or walnuts, and crumbled goat cheese.

7. Drizzle the dressing over the salad ingredients and toss until everything is well coated.

8. Garnish the Roasted Butternut Squash Salad with chopped fresh parsley or cilantro.

9. Serve the salad warm or at room temperature, and enjoy!

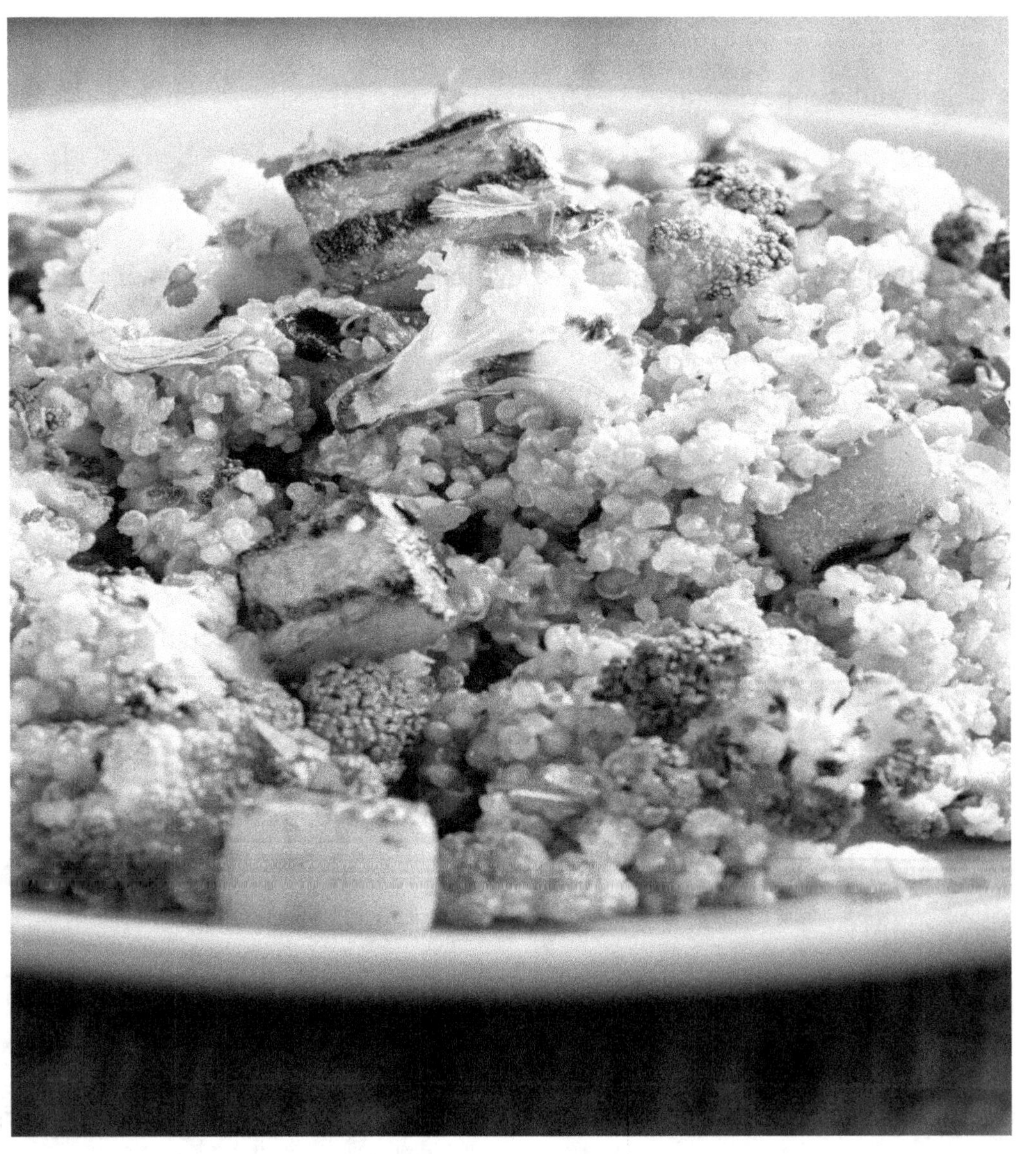

Chapter 10: Salad Recipes

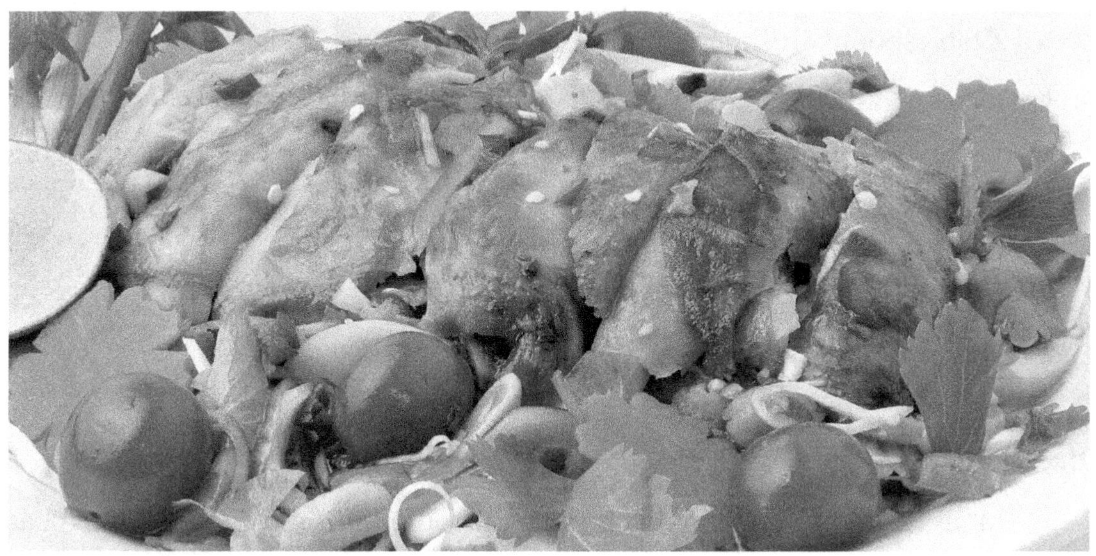

Mediterranean Chickpea Salad with Lemon Herb Dressing

Ingredients:

For the Salad:

- 2 cans (15 ounces each) chickpeas, drained and rinsed
- 1 cup cherry tomatoes, halved
- 1 English cucumber, diced
- 1/2 red onion, finely chopped
- 1/2 cup Kalamata olives, pitted and halved
- 1/4 cup chopped fresh parsley
- 1/4 cup chopped fresh basil
- 1/4 cup crumbled feta cheese (optional)
- Salt and pepper to taste

For the Lemon Herb Dressing:

- 1/4 cup extra virgin olive oil
- 2 tablespoons fresh lemon juice
- 1 clove garlic, minced
- 1 teaspoon Dijon mustard
- 1 teaspoon honey or maple syrup
- 1 tablespoon chopped fresh parsley
- 1 tablespoon chopped fresh basil
- Salt and pepper to taste

Directions:

1. In a large mixing bowl, combine the drained and rinsed chickpeas, cherry tomatoes, diced cucumber, finely chopped red onion, halved Kalamata olives, chopped fresh parsley, and chopped fresh basil. Toss gently to combine.
2. In a small bowl or jar, whisk together the extra virgin olive oil, fresh lemon juice, minced garlic, Dijon mustard, honey or maple syrup, chopped fresh parsley, chopped fresh basil, salt, and pepper until well combined.
3. Pour the Lemon Herb Dressing over the salad ingredients in the mixing bowl. Toss gently until everything is evenly coated with the dressing.
4. If using, sprinkle the crumbled feta cheese over the top of the salad.
5. Taste and adjust seasoning with salt and pepper if needed.
6. Serve the Mediterranean Chickpea Salad with Lemon Herb Dressing immediately, or refrigerate for 30 minutes to allow the flavors to meld together before serving.
7. Enjoy your delicious and nutritious salad!

Spicy Thai Peanut Chicken Salad with Crunchy Vegetables

Ingredients:

For the Salad:

- 2 boneless, skinless chicken breasts
- 6 cups mixed salad greens (such as romaine lettuce, spinach, and cabbage)
- 1 red bell pepper, thinly sliced
- 1 cucumber, julienned
- 1 carrot, julienned
- 1/4 cup chopped cilantro
- 1/4 cup chopped peanuts
- 2 green onions, sliced
- Lime wedges for serving

For the Thai Peanut Dressing:

- 1/4 cup peanut butter (natural, unsweetened)
- 2 tablespoons soy sauce (low-sodium)
- 1 tablespoon rice vinegar
- 1 tablespoon honey or maple syrup
- 1 tablespoon fresh lime juice
- 1 teaspoon sesame oil
- 1 teaspoon grated fresh ginger
- 1 clove garlic, minced
- 1/4 teaspoon red pepper flakes (adjust to taste)
- 2-3 tablespoons water (to thin the dressing)

Directions:

1. Preheat the grill or a grill pan over medium-high heat. Season the chicken breasts with salt and pepper. Grill the chicken for 6-8 minutes per side, or until cooked through and no longer pink in the center. Once cooked, set aside to cool.

2. While the chicken is cooking, prepare the salad ingredients. In a large salad bowl, combine the mixed salad greens, sliced red bell pepper, julienned cucumber, julienned carrot, chopped cilantro, chopped peanuts, and sliced green onions.

3. In a small bowl, whisk together all the ingredients for the Thai Peanut Dressing until smooth. Adjust the consistency by adding more water if needed.

4. Once the chicken has cooled slightly, slice it thinly against the grain.

5. Add the sliced chicken to the salad bowl with the vegetables.

6. Drizzle the Thai Peanut Dressing over the salad, tossing gently to coat everything evenly.

7. Serve the Spicy Thai Peanut Chicken Salad with Crunchy Vegetables immediately, garnished with additional chopped peanuts and cilantro if desired. Serve with lime wedges on the side.

8. Enjoy your delicious and nutritious salad!

Summer Berry and Quinoa Salad with Balsamic Vinaigrette

Ingredients:

For the Salad:

- 1 cup cooked quinoa, cooled

- 2 cups mixed salad greens (such as baby spinach, arugula, or spring mix)
- 1 cup mixed berries (such as strawberries, blueberries, raspberries, and blackberries)
- 1/4 cup sliced almonds, toasted
- 1/4 cup crumbled feta cheese (optional)
- Fresh mint leaves for garnish (optional)

For the Balsamic Vinaigrette:

- 3 tablespoons extra virgin olive oil
- 2 tablespoons balsamic vinegar
- 1 teaspoon Dijon mustard
- 1 teaspoon honey or maple syrup
- Salt and pepper to taste

Directions:

1. In a large salad bowl, combine the cooked quinoa, mixed salad greens, mixed berries, toasted sliced almonds, and crumbled feta cheese (if using). Toss gently to combine.
2. In a small bowl or jar, whisk together the extra virgin olive oil, balsamic vinegar, Dijon mustard, honey or maple syrup, salt, and pepper until well combined.
3. Drizzle the Balsamic Vinaigrette over the salad ingredients in the bowl.
4. Toss the salad gently until everything is evenly coated with the dressing.
5. Garnish the Summer Berry and Quinoa Salad with fresh mint leaves if desired.
6. Serve immediately and enjoy!

Salmon Nicoise Salad with Green Beans and Hard-Boiled Eggs

Ingredients:

For the Salad:

- 2 salmon filets (about 6 ounces each)
- 6 cups mixed salad greens (such as baby spinach, arugula, or spring mix)
- 1 cup cherry tomatoes, halved
- 1/2 cup Niçoise olives, pitted
- 1/2 cup thinly sliced red onion
- 1 cup green beans, blanched
- 4 hard-boiled eggs, peeled and halved
- 1/4 cup chopped fresh parsley (for garnish)
- Lemon wedges for serving

For the Dressing:

- 1/4 cup extra virgin olive oil
- 2 tablespoons red wine vinegar
- 1 tablespoon Dijon mustard
- 1 clove garlic, minced
- Salt and pepper to taste

Directions:

1. Preheat your oven to 400°F (200°C). Place the salmon filets on a baking sheet lined with parchment paper. Drizzle with olive oil and season with salt and pepper. Bake for 12-15 minutes, or until the salmon is cooked through and flakes easily with a fork. Remove from the oven and let it cool slightly.

2. While the salmon is baking, prepare the other salad ingredients. Blanch the green beans in boiling water for 2-3 minutes, then immediately transfer to a bowl of ice water to stop the cooking process. Drain and set aside.

3. Arrange the mixed salad greens on a large serving platter. Top with halved cherry tomatoes, Niçoise olives, thinly sliced red onion, blanched green beans, and halved hard-boiled eggs.

4. Once the salmon has cooled slightly, flake it into large chunks and arrange it on top of the salad.

5. In a small bowl or jar, whisk together the extra virgin olive oil, red wine vinegar, Dijon mustard, minced garlic, salt, and pepper until well combined.

6. Drizzle the dressing over the Salmon Niçoise Salad.

7. Garnish the salad with chopped fresh parsley and serve with lemon wedges on the side.

8. Enjoy your delicious and nutritious Salmon Niçoise Salad with Green Beans and Hard-Boiled Eggs!

Lentil and Arugula Salad with Lemon Garlic Dressing

Ingredients:

For the Salad:

- 1 cup dried green lentils
- 4 cups water or vegetable broth
- 6 cups fresh arugula
- 1/2 cup cherry tomatoes, halved
- 1/4 cup chopped red onion

- 1/4 cup crumbled feta cheese (optional)
- 1/4 cup chopped fresh parsley
- Salt and pepper to taste

For the Lemon Garlic Dressing:

- 1/4 cup extra virgin olive oil
- 2 tablespoons fresh lemon juice
- 1 clove garlic, minced
- 1 teaspoon Dijon mustard
- 1 teaspoon honey or maple syrup
- Salt and pepper to taste

Directions:

1. Rinse the lentils under cold water. In a medium saucepan, combine the rinsed lentils and water or vegetable broth. Bring to a boil, then reduce the heat to low, cover, and simmer for 20-25 minutes, or until the lentils are tender but still hold their shape. Drain any excess liquid and let the lentils cool slightly.

2. In a large salad bowl, combine the cooked lentils, fresh arugula, halved cherry tomatoes, chopped red onion, crumbled feta cheese (if using), and chopped fresh parsley. Toss gently to combine.

3. In a small bowl or jar, whisk together the extra virgin olive oil, fresh lemon juice, minced garlic, Dijon mustard, honey or maple syrup, salt, and pepper until well combined.

4. Drizzle the Lemon Garlic Dressing over the salad ingredients in the bowl.

5. Toss the salad gently until everything is evenly coated with the dressing.

6. Taste and adjust seasoning with salt and pepper if needed.

7. Serve the Lentil and Arugula Salad with Lemon Garlic Dressing immediately, or refrigerate for 30 minutes to allow the flavors to meld together before serving.

8. Enjoy your delicious and nutritious salad!

Southwest Black Bean and Corn Salad with Avocado

Ingredients:

For the Salad:

- 2 cans (15 ounces each) black beans, drained and rinsed
- 1 cup corn kernels (fresh, canned, or thawed if frozen)
- 1 red bell pepper, diced
- 1/2 red onion, finely chopped
- 1 jalapeño pepper, seeded and finely chopped (optional)
- 1 avocado, diced
- 1/4 cup chopped fresh cilantro
- Juice of 2 limes
- Salt and pepper to taste

For the Dressing:

- 3 tablespoons extra virgin olive oil
- 2 tablespoons fresh lime juice
- 1 tablespoon apple cider vinegar
- 1 teaspoon honey or maple syrup
- 1 teaspoon ground cumin
- 1/2 teaspoon chili powder
- 1/4 teaspoon smoked paprika
- Salt and pepper to taste

Directions:

1. In a large salad bowl, combine the black beans, corn kernels, diced red bell pepper, finely chopped red onion, and chopped jalapeño pepper (if using).
2. Add the diced avocado and chopped fresh cilantro to the salad bowl.
3. Squeeze the juice of 2 limes over the salad ingredients.
4. In a small bowl or jar, whisk together the extra virgin olive oil, fresh lime juice, apple cider vinegar, honey or maple syrup, ground cumin, chili powder, smoked paprika, salt, and pepper until well combined.
5. Pour the dressing over the salad ingredients in the bowl.
6. Gently toss the salad until everything is evenly coated with the dressing.
7. Taste and adjust seasoning with salt and pepper if needed.
8. Serve the Southwest Black Bean and Corn Salad with Avocado immediately, or refrigerate for 30 minutes to allow the flavors to meld together before serving.
9. Enjoy your delicious and nutritious salad!

Roasted Beet and Goat Cheese Salad with Mixed Greens

Ingredients:

For the Salad:

- 3 medium beets, trimmed and scrubbed
- 6 cups mixed salad greens (such as baby spinach, arugula, and spring mix)
- 1/2 cup crumbled goat cheese
- 1/4 cup chopped walnuts or pecans, toasted
- 1/4 cup dried cranberries or cherries

- Salt and pepper to taste

For the Balsamic Vinaigrette:

- 1/4 cup extra virgin olive oil
- 2 tablespoons balsamic vinegar
- 1 teaspoon Dijon mustard
- 1 teaspoon honey or maple syrup
- 1 clove garlic, minced
- Salt and pepper to taste

Directions:

1. Preheat your oven to 400°F (200°C). Wrap each beet individually in aluminum foil and place them on a baking sheet. Roast the beets in the preheated oven for 45-60 minutes, or until they are fork-tender. Remove from the oven and let them cool slightly.

2. Once the beets are cool enough to handle, peel off the skin using your fingers or a small knife. Cut the roasted beets into bite-sized wedges or slices.

3. In a large salad bowl, combine the mixed salad greens, roasted beet wedges or slices, crumbled goat cheese, toasted chopped walnuts or pecans, and dried cranberries or cherries. Toss gently to combine.

4. In a small bowl or jar, whisk together the extra virgin olive oil, balsamic vinegar, Dijon mustard, honey or maple syrup, minced garlic, salt, and pepper until well combined.

5. Drizzle the Balsamic Vinaigrette over the salad ingredients in the bowl.

6. Toss the salad gently until everything is evenly coated with the dressing.

7. Taste and adjust seasoning with salt and pepper if needed.

8. Serve the Roasted Beet and Goat Cheese Salad with Mixed Greens immediately, and enjoy!

Greek Chicken Salad with Cucumber and Feta Cheese

Ingredients:

For the Salad:

- 2 boneless, skinless chicken breasts
- 6 cups mixed salad greens (such as romaine lettuce, spinach, and arugula)
- 1 cucumber, diced
- 1 cup cherry tomatoes, halved
- 1/2 red onion, thinly sliced
- 1/4 cup Kalamata olives, pitted and halved
- 1/4 cup crumbled feta cheese
- 2 tablespoons chopped fresh parsley
- Lemon wedges for serving

For the Greek Dressing:

- 1/4 cup extra virgin olive oil
- 2 tablespoons red wine vinegar
- 1 clove garlic, minced
- 1 teaspoon dried oregano
- Salt and pepper to taste

Directions:

1. Preheat your grill or grill pan over medium-high heat. Season the chicken breasts with salt, pepper, and dried oregano. Grill the chicken for 6-8 minutes per side, or until cooked through and no longer pink in the center. Remove from the grill and let them rest for a few minutes before slicing.

2. While the chicken is grilling, prepare the salad ingredients. In a large salad bowl, combine the mixed salad greens, diced cucumber, halved cherry tomatoes, thinly sliced red onion, halved Kalamata olives, crumbled feta cheese, and chopped fresh parsley.

3. In a small bowl or jar, whisk together the extra virgin olive oil, red wine vinegar, minced garlic, dried oregano, salt, and pepper until well combined.

4. Once the chicken has rested, slice it thinly against the grain.

5. Add the sliced chicken to the salad bowl with the vegetables.

6. Drizzle the Greek Dressing over the salad ingredients.

7. Toss the salad gently until everything is evenly coated with the dressing.

8. Serve the Greek Chicken Salad with Cucumber and Feta Cheese immediately, garnished with lemon wedges on the side.

Asian Noodle Salad with Chicken and Vegetables

Ingredients:

For the Salad:

- 8 oz (about 225g) whole wheat spaghetti or soba noodles
- 2 boneless, skinless chicken breasts
- 2 cups shredded cabbage (green or purple)
- 1 red bell pepper, thinly sliced
- 1 carrot, julienned
- 1 cucumber, julienned
- 1/4 cup chopped green onions
- 1/4 cup chopped fresh cilantro
- Sesame seeds for garnish (optional)

For the Dressing:

- 1/4 cup soy sauce (low-sodium)
- 2 tablespoons rice vinegar
- 2 tablespoons sesame oil
- 1 tablespoon honey or maple syrup
- 1 clove garlic, minced
- 1 teaspoon grated fresh ginger
- 1 tablespoon lime juice
- Salt and pepper to taste

Directions:

1. Cook the noodles according to the package instructions until al dente. Drain and rinse under cold water to stop the cooking process. Set aside.

2. Season the chicken breasts with salt and pepper. Heat a grill pan or skillet over medium-high heat and cook the chicken for 6-8 minutes per side, or until cooked through and no longer pink in the center. Remove from the pan and let it rest for a few minutes before slicing thinly.

3. In a large salad bowl, combine the cooked noodles, shredded cabbage, thinly sliced red bell pepper, julienned carrot, julienned cucumber, chopped green onions, and chopped fresh cilantro.

4. In a small bowl, whisk together the soy sauce, rice vinegar, sesame oil, honey or maple syrup, minced garlic, grated ginger, lime juice, salt, and pepper to make the dressing.

5. Pour the dressing over the salad ingredients in the bowl.

6. Toss the salad gently until everything is evenly coated with the dressing.

7. Top the salad with the sliced grilled chicken.

8. Garnish with sesame seeds if desired.

9. Serve the Asian Noodle Salad with Chicken and Vegetables immediately, or refrigerate for 30 minutes to allow the flavors to meld together before serving.

Salmon and Avocado Salad with Whole-Wheat Toast

Ingredients:

For the Salad:

- 2 salmon filets
- 6 cups mixed salad greens (such as spinach, arugula, and romaine)
- 1 avocado, sliced
- 1/2 cup cherry tomatoes, halved
- 1/4 cup sliced red onion
- 1/4 cup chopped cucumber
- 1/4 cup chopped fresh cilantro or parsley
- Lemon wedges for serving

For the Dressing:

- 3 tablespoons extra virgin olive oil
- 2 tablespoons fresh lemon juice
- 1 clove garlic, minced
- 1 teaspoon Dijon mustard
- Salt and pepper to taste

For the Whole-Wheat Toast:

- 4 slices whole-wheat bread
- 1 tablespoon olive oil or butter (optional)

Directions:

1. Preheat your grill or grill pan over medium-high heat. Season the salmon filets with salt and pepper. Grill the salmon for 4-5 minutes per side, or until cooked through and flaky. Remove from the grill and let them rest for a few minutes.

2. While the salmon is grilling, prepare the salad ingredients. In a large salad bowl, combine the mixed salad greens, sliced avocado, halved cherry tomatoes, sliced red onion, chopped cucumber, and chopped fresh cilantro or parsley.

3. In a small bowl or jar, whisk together the extra virgin olive oil, fresh lemon juice, minced garlic, Dijon mustard, salt, and pepper to make the dressing.

4. Drizzle the dressing over the salad ingredients in the bowl.

5. Gently toss the salad until everything is evenly coated with the dressing.

6. Toast the whole-wheat bread slices until golden brown. You can toast them in a toaster or on a grill pan with a little olive oil or butter if desired.

7. Serve the grilled salmon on top of the salad, along with the whole-wheat toast slices and lemon wedges on the side.

8. Enjoy your delicious and nutritious Salmon and Avocado Salad with Whole-Wheat Toast!

Quinoa and Black Bean Salad with Mango and Lime

Ingredients:

For the Salad:

- 1 cup quinoa, rinsed

- 2 cups water or vegetable broth
- 1 can (15 ounces) black beans, drained and rinsed
- 1 ripe mango, diced
- 1 red bell pepper, diced
- 1/4 cup chopped red onion
- 1/4 cup chopped fresh cilantro
- Salt and pepper to taste

For the Dressing:
- 3 tablespoons extra virgin olive oil
- 2 tablespoons fresh lime juice
- 1 teaspoon lime zest
- 1 teaspoon honey or maple syrup
- 1/2 teaspoon ground cumin
- Salt and pepper to taste

Directions:
1. In a medium saucepan, combine the rinsed quinoa and water or vegetable broth. Bring to a boil, then reduce the heat to low, cover, and simmer for 15-20 minutes, or until the quinoa is cooked and the liquid is absorbed. Remove from heat and let it cool slightly.
2. In a large salad bowl, combine the cooked quinoa, black beans, diced mango, diced red bell pepper, chopped red onion, and chopped fresh cilantro.
3. In a small bowl or jar, whisk together the extra virgin olive oil, fresh lime juice, lime zest, honey or maple syrup, ground cumin, salt, and pepper until well combined.
4. Pour the dressing over the salad ingredients in the bowl.
5. Toss the salad gently until everything is evenly coated with the dressing.

6. Taste and adjust seasoning with salt and pepper if needed.

7. Serve the Quinoa and Black Bean Salad with Mango and Lime immediately, or refrigerate for 30 minutes to allow the flavors to meld together before serving.

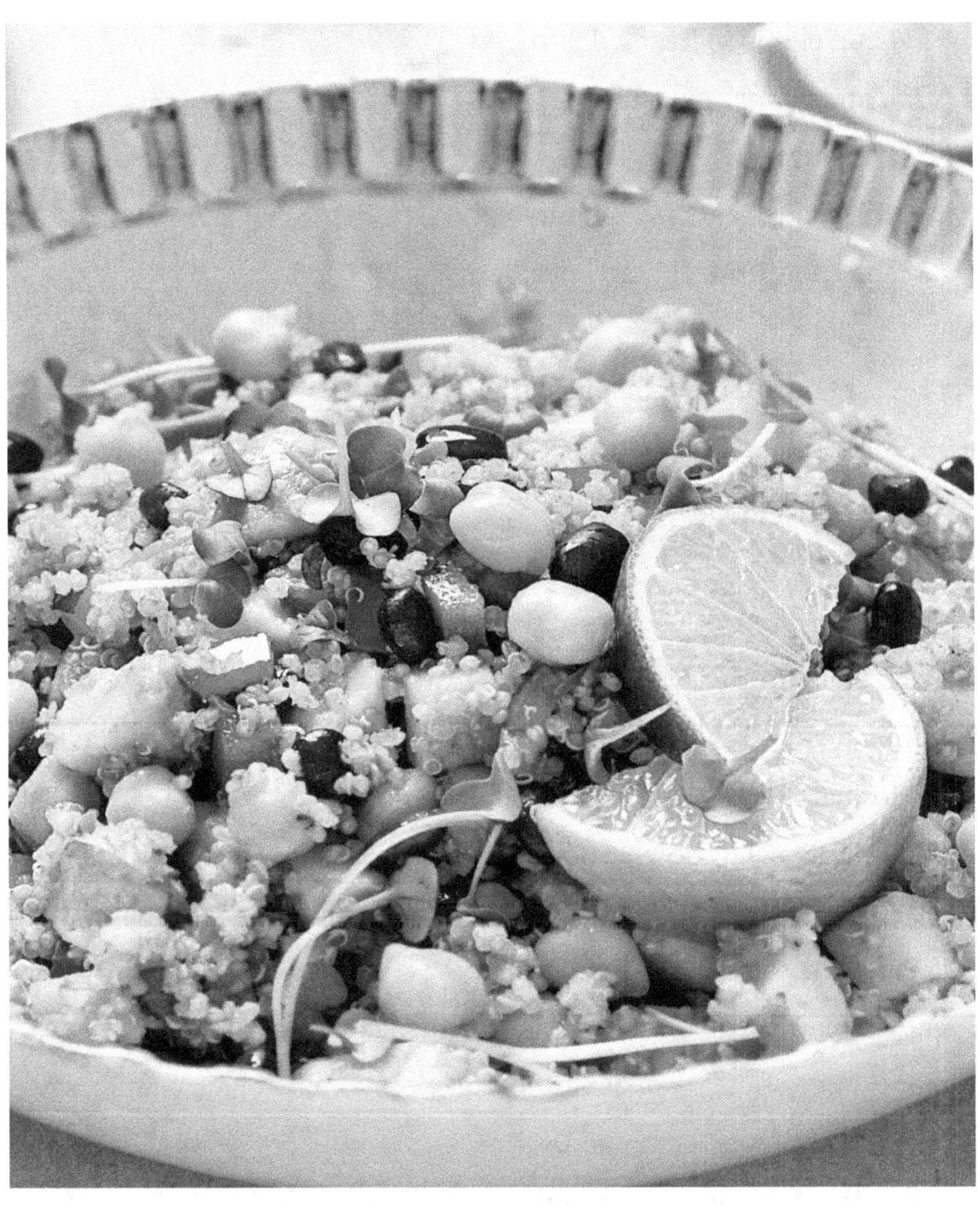

Chapter 11: Soup and Stew Recipes

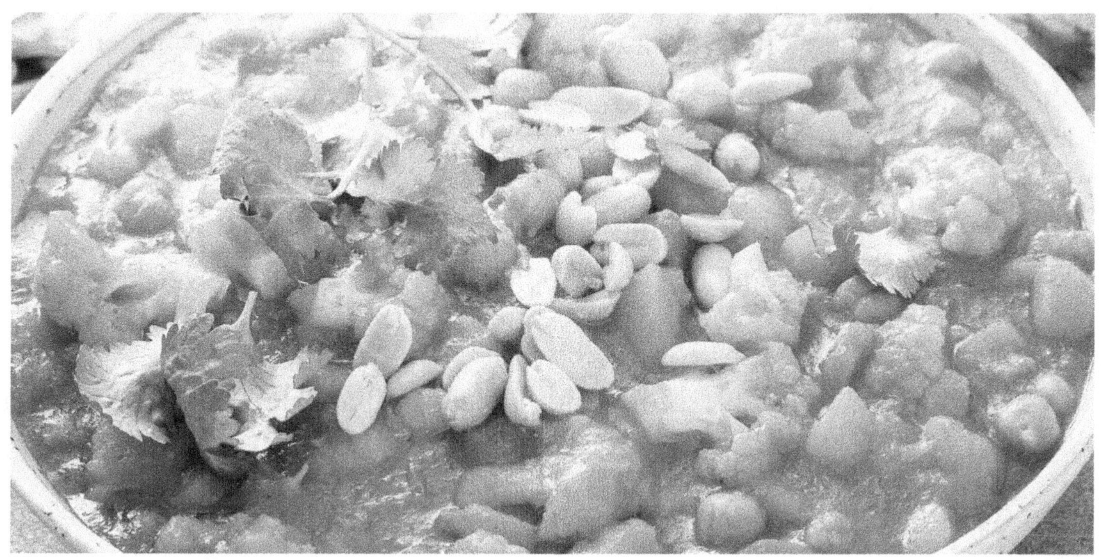

Curried Butternut Squash Soup with Coconut Milk and Chickpeas

Ingredients:

- 1 medium butternut squash, peeled, seeded, and cubed (about 4 cups)
- 1 tablespoon olive oil
- 1 onion, chopped
- 2 cloves garlic, minced
- 1 tablespoon curry powder
- 1 teaspoon ground cumin
- 1/2 teaspoon ground ginger
- 4 cups vegetable broth (low-sodium)
- 1 can (14 ounces) coconut milk (light or full-fat)
- 1 can (15 ounces) chickpeas, drained and rinsed
- Salt and pepper to taste

- Fresh cilantro or parsley for garnish (optional)

Directions:

1. Heat the olive oil in a large pot over medium heat. Add the chopped onion and cook until softened, about 5 minutes.

2. Add the minced garlic, curry powder, ground cumin, and ground ginger to the pot. Cook for 1-2 minutes, stirring constantly, until fragrant.

3. Add the cubed butternut squash to the pot and stir to coat with the spices. Cook for another 5 minutes, stirring occasionally.

4. Pour in the vegetable broth and coconut milk. Bring the mixture to a boil, then reduce the heat to low and let it simmer for 20-25 minutes, or until the butternut squash is tender.

5. Once the butternut squash is cooked, use an immersion blender to blend the soup until smooth and creamy. Alternatively, you can carefully transfer the soup to a blender in batches and blend until smooth, then return it to the pot.

6. Stir in the drained and rinsed chickpeas and simmer for another 5 minutes to heat through.

7. Season the soup with salt and pepper to taste.

8. Serve the Curried Butternut Squash Soup with Coconut Milk and Chickpeas hot, garnished with fresh cilantro or parsley if desired.

Thai Coconut Curry Chicken Stew with Vegetables and Brown Rice

Ingredients:

For the Stew:

- 1 tablespoon coconut oil
- 1 onion, diced

- 2 cloves garlic, minced

- 1 tablespoon grated fresh ginger

- 1 red bell pepper, sliced

- 1 yellow bell pepper, sliced

- 2 carrots, sliced

- 1 zucchini, sliced

- 1 pound boneless, skinless chicken breasts, cut into bite-sized pieces

- 2 tablespoons Thai red curry paste

- 1 can (14 ounces) coconut milk (light or full-fat)

- 2 cups low-sodium chicken broth

- 2 tablespoons fish sauce (optional)

- 1 tablespoon soy sauce (low-sodium)

- 1 tablespoon brown sugar or coconut sugar

- Juice of 1 lime

- Salt and pepper to taste

- Fresh cilantro for garnish (optional)

For the Brown Rice:

- 1 cup brown rice

- 2 cups water or low-sodium chicken broth

Directions:

1. In a large pot or Dutch oven, heat the coconut oil over medium heat. Add the diced onion and cook until softened, about 5 minutes.

2. Add the minced garlic and grated ginger to the pot, and cook for another 1-2 minutes, stirring constantly, until fragrant.

3. Add the sliced red bell pepper, yellow bell pepper, carrots, and zucchini to the pot. Cook for 5 minutes, stirring occasionally, until the vegetables are slightly softened.

4. Push the vegetables to one side of the pot and add the chicken pieces to the empty side. Cook for 5-7 minutes, stirring occasionally, until the chicken is browned on all sides.

5. Stir in the Thai red curry paste and cook for 1 minute, stirring constantly, until fragrant.

6. Pour in the coconut milk, chicken broth, fish sauce (if using), soy sauce, and brown sugar. Stir to combine.

7. Bring the stew to a simmer, then reduce the heat to low and let it simmer for 20-25 minutes, or until the chicken is cooked through and the vegetables are tender.

8. While the stew is simmering, prepare the brown rice. Rinse the brown rice under cold water, then combine it with water or chicken broth in a medium saucepan. Bring to a boil, then reduce the heat to low, cover, and simmer for 40-45 minutes, or until the rice is tender and the liquid is absorbed.

9. Once the stew is ready, stir in the lime juice and season with salt and pepper to taste.

10. Serve the Thai Coconut Curry Chicken Stew with Vegetables over cooked brown rice, garnished with fresh cilantro if desired.

Minestrone Soup with Whole-Wheat Bread

Ingredients:

For the Soup:
- 1 tablespoon olive oil
- 1 onion, diced
- 2 cloves garlic, minced
- 2 carrots, diced

- 2 celery stalks, diced

- 1 zucchini, diced

- 1 yellow squash, diced

- 1 can (14 ounces) diced tomatoes

- 6 cups low-sodium vegetable broth

- 1 can (15 ounces) kidney beans, drained and rinsed

- 1 can (15 ounces) cannellini beans, drained and rinsed

- 1 cup chopped fresh spinach or kale

- 1 teaspoon dried oregano

- 1 teaspoon dried basil

- Salt and pepper to taste

- Grated Parmesan cheese for serving (optional)

For the Whole-Wheat Bread:

- 4 slices whole-wheat bread

- 1 tablespoon olive oil or butter (optional)

Directions:

1. In a large pot or Dutch oven, heat the olive oil over medium heat. Add the diced onion and cook until softened, about 5 minutes.

2. Add the minced garlic to the pot and cook for another 1-2 minutes, stirring constantly, until fragrant.

3. Add the diced carrots, celery, zucchini, and yellow squash to the pot. Cook for 5 minutes, stirring occasionally, until the vegetables start to soften.

4. Pour in the diced tomatoes and vegetable broth. Bring the mixture to a boil, then reduce the heat to low and let it simmer for 15-20 minutes, or until the vegetables are tender.

5. Stir in the drained and rinsed kidney beans, cannellini beans, chopped spinach or kale, dried oregano, and dried basil. Simmer for another 5-10 minutes to heat through.

6. While the soup is simmering, prepare the whole-wheat bread. You can toast the bread slices in a toaster or on a grill pan with a little olive oil or butter if desired.

7. Season the soup with salt and pepper to taste.

8. Serve the Minestrone Soup hot, garnished with grated Parmesan cheese if desired, and accompanied by whole-wheat bread slices.

Spicy Lentil Soup with Whole-Wheat Pita Bread

Ingredients:

For the Soup:

- 1 tablespoon olive oil
- 1 onion, diced
- 2 cloves garlic, minced
- 2 carrots, diced
- 2 celery stalks, diced
- 1 red bell pepper, diced
- 1 cup dried brown lentils, rinsed and drained
- 1 can (14 ounces) diced tomatoes
- 6 cups low-sodium vegetable broth
- 1 teaspoon ground cumin
- 1 teaspoon ground coriander
- 1/2 teaspoon smoked paprika
- 1/4 teaspoon cayenne pepper (adjust to taste)
- Salt and pepper to taste

- Fresh cilantro or parsley for garnish (optional)

For the Whole-Wheat Pita Bread:

- 4 whole-wheat pita bread rounds

Directions:

1. In a large pot or Dutch oven, heat the olive oil over medium heat. Add the diced onion and cook until softened, about 5 minutes.

2. Add the minced garlic to the pot and cook for another 1-2 minutes, stirring constantly, until fragrant.

3. Add the diced carrots, celery, and red bell pepper to the pot. Cook for 5 minutes, stirring occasionally, until the vegetables start to soften.

4. Stir in the rinsed and drained brown lentils, diced tomatoes, vegetable broth, ground cumin, ground coriander, smoked paprika, and cayenne pepper.

5. Bring the soup to a boil, then reduce the heat to low and let it simmer for 25-30 minutes, or until the lentils are tender.

6. While the soup is simmering, preheat the oven to 350°F (175°C). Place the whole-wheat pita bread rounds on a baking sheet and bake for 5-7 minutes, or until warm and slightly crispy.

7. Season the soup with salt and pepper to taste.

8. Serve the Spicy Lentil Soup hot, garnished with fresh cilantro or parsley if desired, and accompanied by whole-wheat pita bread rounds.

Creamy Tomato Tortilla Soup with a dollop of Greek Yogurt

Ingredients:

- 1 tablespoon olive oil
- 1 onion, diced

- 2 cloves garlic, minced
- 1 red bell pepper, diced
- 1 can (14 ounces) diced tomatoes
- 2 cups low-sodium vegetable broth
- 1 teaspoon ground cumin
- 1 teaspoon smoked paprika
- 1/2 teaspoon chili powder
- Salt and pepper to taste
- 1/2 cup plain Greek yogurt
- 4 whole-grain tortillas, cut into strips
- Fresh cilantro for garnish (optional)
- Lime wedges for serving (optional)

Directions:

1. In a large pot or Dutch oven, heat the olive oil over medium heat. Add the diced onion and cook until softened, about 5 minutes.

2. Add the minced garlic to the pot and cook for another 1-2 minutes, stirring constantly, until fragrant.

3. Add the diced red bell pepper to the pot and cook for 5 minutes, stirring occasionally, until softened.

4. Stir in the diced tomatoes, vegetable broth, ground cumin, smoked paprika, and chili powder. Bring the soup to a boil, then reduce the heat to low and let it simmer for 15-20 minutes, stirring occasionally.

5. While the soup is simmering, preheat the oven to 350°F (175°C). Place the tortilla strips on a baking sheet and bake for 8-10 minutes, or until crisp and golden brown.

6. Use an immersion blender to blend the soup until smooth and creamy. Alternatively, you can carefully transfer the soup to a blender in batches and blend until smooth, then return it to the pot.

7. Season the soup with salt and pepper to taste.

8. Ladle the Creamy Tomato Tortilla Soup into bowls. Top each serving with a dollop of Greek yogurt and a handful of baked tortilla strips.

9. Garnish with fresh cilantro and serve with lime wedges on the side for squeezing over the soup, if desired.

Split Pea Soup with Whole-Wheat Crackers

Ingredients:

- 1 tablespoon olive oil
- 1 onion, diced
- 2 carrots, diced
- 2 celery stalks, diced
- 2 cloves garlic, minced
- 1 bay leaf
- 1 teaspoon dried thyme
- 1 teaspoon dried rosemary
- 1 pound dried split peas, rinsed and drained
- 6 cups low-sodium vegetable broth or water
- Salt and pepper to taste
- Fresh parsley for garnish (optional)
- Whole-wheat crackers for serving

Directions:

1. In a large pot or Dutch oven, heat the olive oil over medium heat. Add the diced onion, carrots, and celery to the pot. Cook for 5-7 minutes, stirring occasionally, until the vegetables start to soften.

2. Add the minced garlic, bay leaf, dried thyme, and dried rosemary to the pot. Cook for another 1-2 minutes, stirring constantly, until fragrant.

3. Stir in the rinsed and drained split peas and vegetable broth or water. Bring the mixture to a boil, then reduce the heat to low and let it simmer for 45-60 minutes, or until the split peas are soft and tender, stirring occasionally.

4. Once the split peas are cooked, use an immersion blender to blend the soup until smooth and creamy. Alternatively, you can carefully transfer the soup to a blender in batches and blend until smooth, then return it to the pot.

5. Season the soup with salt and pepper to taste.

6. Ladle the Split Pea Soup into bowls. Garnish with fresh parsley if desired, and serve with whole-wheat crackers on the side.

Vegetable Barley Soup with Parmesan Cheese Rind

Ingredients:

- 1 tablespoon olive oil
- 1 onion, diced
- 2 carrots, diced
- 2 celery stalks, diced
- 2 cloves garlic, minced
- 1 can (14 ounces) diced tomatoes

- 1/2 cup pearl barley, rinsed and drained
- 6 cups low-sodium vegetable broth or water
- 1 Parmesan cheese rind (about 2 inches)
- 2 bay leaves
- 1 teaspoon dried thyme
- Salt and pepper to taste
- Grated Parmesan cheese for serving (optional)
- Fresh parsley for garnish (optional)

Directions:

1. In a large pot or Dutch oven, heat the olive oil over medium heat. Add the diced onion, carrots, and celery to the pot. Cook for 5-7 minutes, stirring occasionally, until the vegetables start to soften.
2. Add the minced garlic to the pot and cook for another 1-2 minutes, stirring constantly, until fragrant.
3. Stir in the diced tomatoes, rinsed and drained pearl barley, vegetable broth or water, Parmesan cheese rind, bay leaves, and dried thyme.
4. Bring the soup to a boil, then reduce the heat to low and let it simmer for 45-60 minutes, or until the barley is tender and cooked through, stirring occasionally.
5. Once the barley is cooked, remove the Parmesan cheese rind and bay leaves from the soup. Season the soup with salt and pepper to taste.
6. Ladle the Vegetable Barley Soup into bowls. Serve hot, garnished with grated Parmesan cheese and fresh parsley if desired.

French Lentil Stew with Whole-Wheat Bread

Ingredients:

- 1 tablespoon olive oil

- 1 onion, diced
- 2 carrots, diced
- 2 celery stalks, diced
- 2 cloves garlic, minced
- 1 cup French green lentils, rinsed and drained
- 4 cups low-sodium vegetable broth or water
- 1 can (14 ounces) diced tomatoes
- 2 bay leaves
- 1 teaspoon dried thyme
- Salt and pepper to taste
- Fresh parsley for garnish (optional)
- Whole-wheat bread slices for serving

Directions:

1. In a large pot or Dutch oven, heat the olive oil over medium heat. Add the diced onion, carrots, and celery to the pot. Cook for 5-7 minutes, stirring occasionally, until the vegetables start to soften.

2. Add the minced garlic to the pot and cook for another 1-2 minutes, stirring constantly, until fragrant.

3. Stir in the rinsed and drained French green lentils, vegetable broth or water, diced tomatoes, bay leaves, and dried thyme.

4. Bring the stew to a boil, then reduce the heat to low and let it simmer for 30-40 minutes, or until the lentils are tender, stirring occasionally.

5. Once the lentils are cooked, remove the bay leaves from the stew. Season the stew with salt and pepper to taste.

6. Ladle the French Lentil Stew into bowls. Serve hot, garnished with fresh parsley if desired, and accompanied by whole-wheat bread slices.

Roasted Poblano and Corn Chowder with a dollop of Low-Fat Sour Cream

Ingredients:

- 2 poblano peppers
- 2 tablespoons olive oil, divided
- 1 onion, diced
- 2 cloves garlic, minced
- 2 potatoes, peeled and diced
- 4 cups low-sodium vegetable broth
- 2 cups frozen corn kernels
- 1 cup low-fat milk or unsweetened almond milk
- Salt and pepper to taste
- Low-fat sour cream for serving
- Fresh cilantro or parsley for garnish (optional)

Directions:

1. Preheat the oven to broil. Place the poblano peppers on a baking sheet and drizzle with 1 tablespoon of olive oil. Broil for 5-7 minutes, turning occasionally, until the peppers are charred and blistered on all sides. Remove from the oven and let cool. Once cooled, remove the skins, seeds, and stems from the peppers, then dice them.

2. In a large pot or Dutch oven, heat the remaining 1 tablespoon of olive oil over medium heat. Add the diced onion and cook for 5-7 minutes, stirring occasionally, until softened.

3. Add the minced garlic to the pot and cook for another 1-2 minutes, stirring constantly, until fragrant.

4. Stir in the diced potatoes and vegetable broth. Bring the mixture to a boil, then reduce the heat to low and let it simmer for 15-20 minutes, or until the potatoes are tender.

5. Once the potatoes are cooked, stir in the diced roasted poblano peppers and frozen corn kernels. Let the soup simmer for another 5 minutes to heat through.

6. Use an immersion blender to blend the soup until smooth and creamy. Alternatively, you can carefully transfer the soup to a blender in batches and blend until smooth, then return it to the pot.

7. Stir in the low-fat milk or unsweetened almond milk. Season the chowder with salt and pepper to taste.

8. Ladle the Roasted Poblano and Corn Chowder into bowls. Top each serving with a dollop of low-fat sour cream and garnish with fresh cilantro or parsley if desired.

Tuscan White Bean Soup with Kale and Cannellini Beans

Ingredients:
- 1 tablespoon olive oil
- 1 onion, diced
- 2 carrots, diced
- 2 celery stalks, diced
- 2 cloves garlic, minced
- 1 teaspoon dried thyme
- 1 teaspoon dried rosemary
- 1 can (15 ounces) cannellini beans, drained and rinsed
- 4 cups low-sodium vegetable broth

- 1 bunch kale, stems removed and leaves chopped

- Salt and pepper to taste

- Grated Parmesan cheese for serving (optional)

Directions:

1. In a large pot or Dutch oven, heat the olive oil over medium heat. Add the diced onion, carrots, and celery to the pot. Cook for 5-7 minutes, stirring occasionally, until the vegetables start to soften.

2. Add the minced garlic, dried thyme, and dried rosemary to the pot. Cook for another 1-2 minutes, stirring constantly, until fragrant.

3. Stir in the drained and rinsed cannellini beans and vegetable broth. Bring the mixture to a boil, then reduce the heat to low and let it simmer for 15-20 minutes, stirring occasionally.

4. Use an immersion blender to blend a portion of the soup until smooth and creamy. This step helps thicken the soup while still leaving some whole beans for texture. Alternatively, you can transfer a portion of the soup to a blender and blend until smooth, then return it to the pot.

5. Stir in the chopped kale leaves and let the soup simmer for another 5-10 minutes, or until the kale is wilted and tender.

6. Season the Tuscan White Bean Soup with salt and pepper to taste.

7. Ladle the soup into bowls and serve hot, optionally topping each serving with grated Parmesan cheese.

Moroccan Chickpea and Vegetable Stew with Couscous

Ingredients:

For the Stew:

- 1 tablespoon olive oil

- 1 onion, diced
- 2 carrots, diced
- 2 celery stalks, diced
- 2 cloves garlic, minced
- 1 teaspoon ground cumin
- 1 teaspoon ground coriander
- 1 teaspoon ground turmeric
- 1/2 teaspoon ground cinnamon
- 1 can (15 ounces) chickpeas, drained and rinsed
- 1 can (14 ounces) diced tomatoes
- 3 cups low-sodium vegetable broth
- 1 cup diced zucchini
- 1 cup diced bell peppers (any color)
- Salt and pepper to taste
- Fresh cilantro for garnish (optional)

For the Couscous:

- 1 cup whole-wheat couscous
- 1 1/4 cups low-sodium vegetable broth
- 1 tablespoon olive oil
- Salt and pepper to taste

Directions:

1. In a large pot or Dutch oven, heat the olive oil over medium heat. Add the diced onion, carrots, and celery to the pot. Cook for 5-7 minutes, stirring occasionally, until the vegetables start to soften.

2. Add the minced garlic, ground cumin, ground coriander, ground turmeric, and ground cinnamon to the pot. Cook for another 1-2 minutes, stirring constantly, until fragrant.

3. Stir in the drained and rinsed chickpeas, diced tomatoes, and low-sodium vegetable broth. Bring the mixture to a boil, then reduce the heat to low and let it simmer for 15-20 minutes.

4. While the stew is simmering, prepare the couscous. In a separate pot, bring the low-sodium vegetable broth and olive oil to a boil. Stir in the whole-wheat couscous, cover the pot, and remove it from the heat. Let the couscous sit for 5 minutes, then fluff it with a fork. Season with salt and pepper to taste.

5. Stir the diced zucchini and bell peppers into the stew. Let it simmer for another 5-10 minutes, or until the vegetables are tender.

6. Season the Moroccan Chickpea and Vegetable Stew with salt and pepper to taste.

7. Serve the stew hot, accompanied by the whole-wheat couscous. Garnish with fresh cilantro if desired.

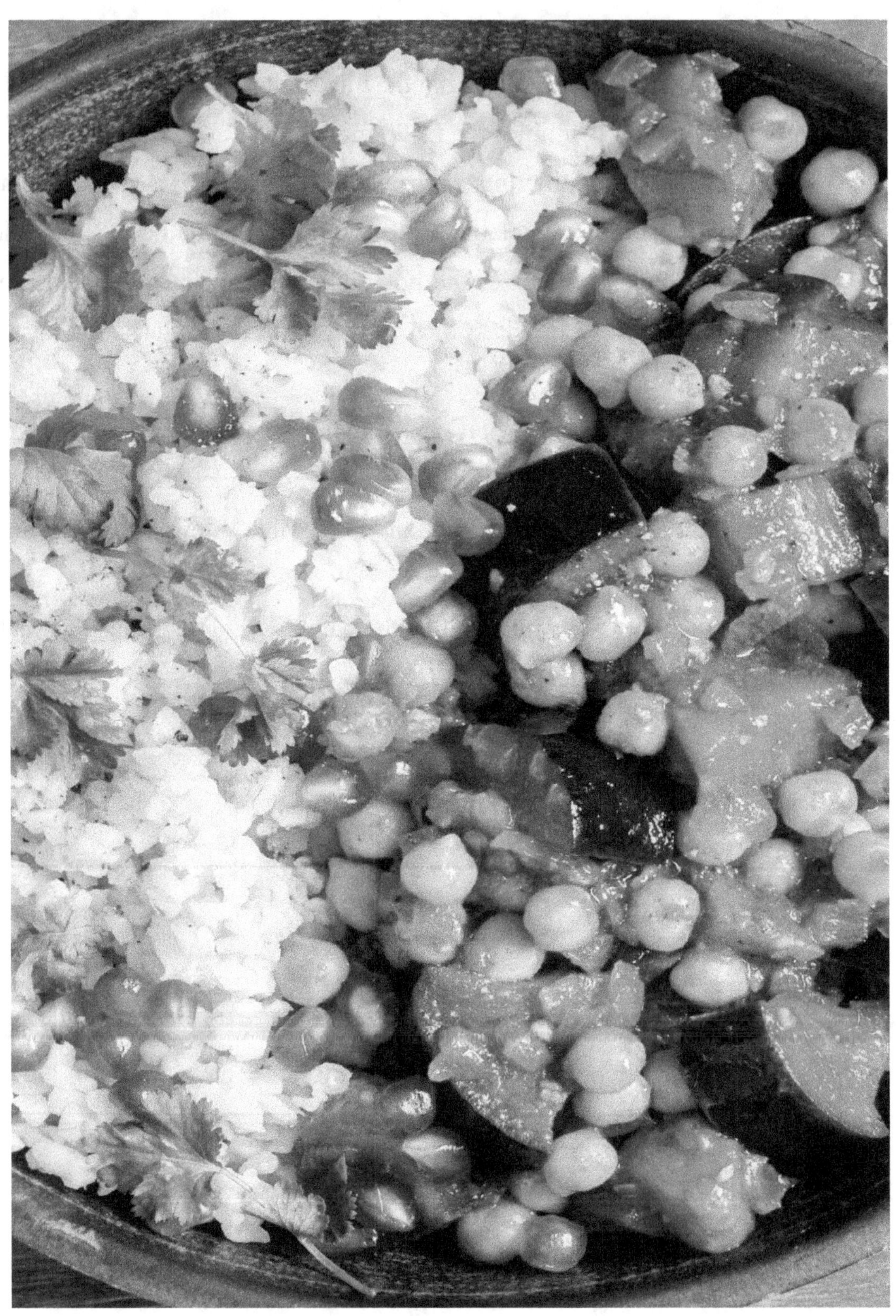

Chapter 12: Meat and Poultry Recipes

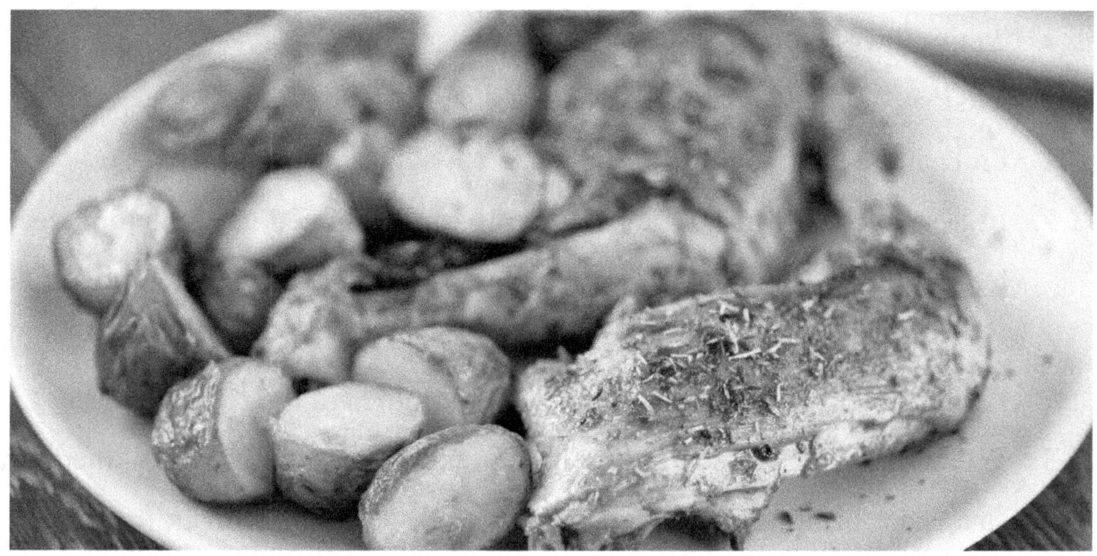

Lemon Garlic Chicken with Roasted Asparagus and Quinoa

Ingredients:

For the Lemon Garlic Chicken:

- 4 boneless, skinless chicken breasts
- 2 tablespoons olive oil
- 3 cloves garlic, minced
- Zest and juice of 1 lemon
- 1 teaspoon dried oregano
- Salt and pepper to taste

For the Roasted Asparagus:

- 1 bunch asparagus, tough ends trimmed
- 1 tablespoon olive oil
- Salt and pepper to taste

For the Quinoa:

- 1 cup quinoa, rinsed
- 2 cups low-sodium chicken broth or water

Directions:

1. Preheat the oven to 400°F (200°C).

2. In a small bowl, mix together the olive oil, minced garlic, lemon zest, lemon juice, dried oregano, salt, and pepper. Place the chicken breasts in a shallow dish and pour the marinade over them, turning to coat evenly. Let the chicken marinate for at least 30 minutes in the refrigerator.

3. While the chicken is marinating, prepare the quinoa. In a medium saucepan, bring the chicken broth or water to a boil. Stir in the quinoa, reduce the heat to low, cover, and simmer for 15-20 minutes, or until the quinoa is tender and the liquid is absorbed. Fluff the quinoa with a fork and set aside.

4. Place the trimmed asparagus spears on a baking sheet. Drizzle with olive oil and season with salt and pepper. Toss to coat evenly. Roast in the preheated oven for 10-12 minutes, or until tender but still crisp.

5. While the asparagus is roasting, heat a grill pan or skillet over medium-high heat. Remove the chicken breasts from the marinade and discard any excess marinade. Cook the chicken breasts for 6-8 minutes per side, or until cooked through and no longer pink in the center.

6. Once the chicken is cooked through, remove it from the heat and let it rest for a few minutes before slicing.

7. To serve, divide the cooked quinoa among plates. Top with sliced lemon garlic chicken and roasted asparagus.

8. Enjoy your delicious and nutritious Lemon Garlic Chicken with Roasted Asparagus and Quinoa!

Turkey Meatloaf Muffins with Mashed Cauliflower

Ingredients:

For the Turkey Meatloaf Muffins:

- 1 lb lean ground turkey
- 1/2 cup rolled oats (or breadcrumbs)
- 1/4 cup grated Parmesan cheese
- 1/4 cup chopped onion
- 1/4 cup chopped bell pepper
- 2 cloves garlic, minced
- 1 egg
- 2 tablespoons tomato paste
- 1 teaspoon Worcestershire sauce
- 1 teaspoon Italian seasoning
- Salt and pepper to taste

For the Mashed Cauliflower:

- 1 head cauliflower, chopped into florets
- 2 cloves garlic, minced
- 1/4 cup low-fat milk or unsweetened almond milk
- 2 tablespoons grated Parmesan cheese
- Salt and pepper to taste

Directions:

1. Preheat the oven to 375°F (190°C). Lightly grease a muffin tin or line with muffin liners.
2. In a large mixing bowl, combine the ground turkey, rolled oats (or breadcrumbs), grated Parmesan cheese, chopped onion, chopped bell pepper, minced garlic, egg, tomato paste, Worcestershire sauce, Italian seasoning, salt, and pepper. Mix until well combined.

3. Divide the turkey mixture evenly among the muffin cups, pressing down gently to form into muffins.

4. Bake the turkey meatloaf muffins in the preheated oven for 20-25 minutes, or until cooked through and lightly browned on top.

5. While the turkey meatloaf muffins are baking, prepare the mashed cauliflower. Place the cauliflower florets in a steamer basket over a pot of boiling water. Steam for 10-12 minutes, or until tender.

6. Transfer the steamed cauliflower to a food processor. Add the minced garlic, low-fat milk or unsweetened almond milk, grated Parmesan cheese, salt, and pepper. Blend until smooth and creamy.

7. Once the turkey meatloaf muffins are done baking, remove them from the oven and let them cool slightly.

8. Serve the turkey meatloaf muffins with a dollop of mashed cauliflower on the side.

9. Enjoy your delicious and nutritious Turkey Meatloaf Muffins with Mashed Cauliflower!

Harissa-Spiced Chicken Thighs with Roasted Sweet Potato Wedges

Ingredients:

For the Harissa-Spiced Chicken Thighs:

- 4 bone-in, skin-on chicken thighs
- 2 tablespoons harissa paste
- 1 tablespoon olive oil
- 2 cloves garlic, minced
- 1 teaspoon ground cumin
- 1 teaspoon smoked paprika

- 1/2 teaspoon ground coriander
- Salt and pepper to taste

For the Roasted Sweet Potato Wedges:

- 2 medium sweet potatoes, washed and cut into wedges
- 1 tablespoon olive oil
- 1 teaspoon smoked paprika
- 1/2 teaspoon garlic powder
- Salt and pepper to taste

Directions:

1. Preheat the oven to 400°F (200°C). Line a baking sheet with parchment paper or foil for easy cleanup.

2. In a small bowl, mix together the harissa paste, olive oil, minced garlic, ground cumin, smoked paprika, ground coriander, salt, and pepper to make the marinade for the chicken thighs.

3. Place the chicken thighs in a shallow dish or resealable plastic bag. Pour the marinade over the chicken thighs, turning to coat evenly. Let the chicken thighs marinate for at least 30 minutes in the refrigerator.

4. While the chicken thighs are marinating, prepare the sweet potato wedges. Place the sweet potato wedges on the prepared baking sheet. Drizzle with olive oil and sprinkle with smoked paprika, garlic powder, salt, and pepper. Toss to coat evenly.

5. Arrange the marinated chicken thighs on the baking sheet alongside the sweet potato wedges.

6. Roast in the preheated oven for 25-30 minutes, or until the chicken thighs are cooked through and the sweet potato wedges are tender and caramelized, flipping the sweet potato wedges halfway through cooking.

7. Once the chicken thighs and sweet potato wedges are done roasting, remove them from the oven and let them rest for a few minutes before serving.

8. Serve the Harissa-Spiced Chicken Thighs with Roasted Sweet Potato Wedges hot, and enjoy!

One-Pan Cajun Shrimp and Sausage with Dirty Rice

Ingredients:

For the Cajun Shrimp and Sausage:

- 1 lb large shrimp, peeled and deveined
- 12 oz Andouille sausage, sliced
- 1 tablespoon olive oil
- 1 onion, diced
- 1 bell pepper, diced
- 2 celery stalks, diced
- 3 cloves garlic, minced
- 1 tablespoon Cajun seasoning
- 1 teaspoon paprika
- 1/2 teaspoon dried thyme
- Salt and pepper to taste
- Fresh parsley for garnish (optional)

For the Dirty Rice:

- 1 cup long-grain white rice
- 2 cups low-sodium chicken broth
- 1 tablespoon olive oil
- 1 onion, diced

- 2 cloves garlic, minced

- 1 bell pepper, diced

- 2 celery stalks, diced

- 1/2 teaspoon dried thyme

- 1/2 teaspoon dried oregano

- 1/2 teaspoon paprika

- Salt and pepper to taste

- Green onions for garnish (optional)

Directions:

1. Start by preparing the dirty rice. In a large skillet or pan, heat 1 tablespoon of olive oil over medium heat. Add the diced onion, bell pepper, and celery to the skillet. Cook for 5-7 minutes, stirring occasionally, until the vegetables start to soften.

2. Stir in the minced garlic, dried thyme, dried oregano, paprika, salt, and pepper. Cook for another 1-2 minutes, until fragrant.

3. Add the rice to the skillet and cook for 1-2 minutes, stirring constantly, until the rice is lightly toasted.

4. Pour the low-sodium chicken broth into the skillet and bring the mixture to a boil. Reduce the heat to low, cover the skillet, and let the rice simmer for 15-20 minutes, or until the liquid is absorbed and the rice is cooked through.

5. While the rice is cooking, prepare the Cajun shrimp and sausage. In a separate large skillet or pan, heat 1 tablespoon of olive oil over medium-high heat. Add the sliced Andouille sausage to the skillet and cook for 3-4 minutes, until browned.

6. Add the diced onion, bell pepper, and celery to the skillet with the sausage. Cook for 5-7 minutes, stirring occasionally, until the vegetables are tender.

7. Stir in the minced garlic, Cajun seasoning, paprika, dried thyme, salt, and pepper. Cook for another 1-2 minutes, until fragrant.

8. Add the peeled and deveined shrimp to the skillet with the sausage and vegetables. Cook for 3-4 minutes, stirring occasionally, until the shrimp are pink and cooked through.

9. Once the rice is done cooking, fluff it with a fork and add it to the skillet with the Cajun shrimp and sausage. Stir everything together until well combined.

10. Serve the One-Pan Cajun Shrimp and Sausage with Dirty Rice hot, garnished with fresh parsley or green onions if desired.

Chicken Stir-Fry with Snow Peas, Mushrooms, and Brown Rice

Ingredients:

For the Chicken Stir-Fry:

- 1 lb boneless, skinless chicken breast, thinly sliced
- 2 tablespoons low-sodium soy sauce
- 1 tablespoon oyster sauce
- 1 tablespoon cornstarch
- 2 tablespoons olive oil, divided
- 2 cloves garlic, minced
- 1 teaspoon grated ginger
- 2 cups snow peas, trimmed
- 8 oz mushrooms, sliced

- 1 bell pepper, thinly sliced

- Salt and pepper to taste

- Crushed red pepper flakes (optional)

For the Brown Rice:

- 1 cup brown rice

- 2 cups water or low-sodium chicken broth

Directions:

1. Start by cooking the brown rice. In a medium saucepan, bring the water or low-sodium chicken broth to a boil. Stir in the brown rice, reduce the heat to low, cover, and simmer for 40-45 minutes, or until the rice is tender and the liquid is absorbed. Remove from heat and let it sit covered for 5 minutes, then fluff with a fork.

2. In a small bowl, whisk together the low-sodium soy sauce, oyster sauce, and cornstarch to make the marinade for the chicken.

3. Place the thinly sliced chicken breast in a shallow dish and pour the marinade over it, tossing to coat evenly. Let the chicken marinate for at least 15 minutes.

4. Heat 1 tablespoon of olive oil in a large skillet or wok over medium-high heat. Add the minced garlic and grated ginger to the skillet and cook for 1 minute, until fragrant.

5. Add the marinated chicken to the skillet and stir-fry for 5-6 minutes, or until cooked through and no longer pink. Remove the chicken from the skillet and set aside.

6. In the same skillet, heat the remaining 1 tablespoon of olive oil over medium-high heat. Add the snow peas, sliced mushrooms, and thinly sliced bell pepper to the skillet. Stir-fry for 3-4 minutes, or until the vegetables are tender-crisp.

7. Return the cooked chicken to the skillet with the vegetables. Season with salt, pepper, and crushed red pepper flakes if desired. Stir everything together and cook for another 1-2 minutes to heat through.

8. Serve the Chicken Stir-Fry with Snow Peas, Mushrooms, and Brown Rice hot, garnished with sliced green onions or sesame seeds if desired.

Baked Chicken Fajitas with Portobello Mushrooms and Whole-Wheat Tortillas

Ingredients:

For the Baked Chicken Fajitas:

- 1 lb boneless, skinless chicken breasts, thinly sliced
- 2 large portobello mushrooms, sliced
- 1 onion, thinly sliced
- 1 red bell pepper, thinly sliced
- 1 green bell pepper, thinly sliced
- 2 tablespoons olive oil
- 2 cloves garlic, minced
- 1 tablespoon chili powder
- 1 teaspoon ground cumin
- 1/2 teaspoon paprika
- 1/2 teaspoon dried oregano
- Salt and pepper to taste
- Juice of 1 lime
- Fresh cilantro for garnish (optional)

For Serving:

- Whole-wheat tortillas
- Sliced avocado

- Greek yogurt or sour cream

- Salsa

Directions:

1. Preheat the oven to 400°F (200°C). Lightly grease a large baking sheet or line it with parchment paper.

2. In a large mixing bowl, combine the thinly sliced chicken breasts, sliced portobello mushrooms, thinly sliced onion, thinly sliced red bell pepper, and thinly sliced green bell pepper.

3. In a small bowl, whisk together the olive oil, minced garlic, chili powder, ground cumin, paprika, dried oregano, salt, pepper, and lime juice.

4. Pour the spice mixture over the chicken and vegetable mixture in the large mixing bowl. Toss to coat everything evenly.

5. Spread the chicken and vegetable mixture out onto the prepared baking sheet in an even layer.

6. Bake in the preheated oven for 20-25 minutes, or until the chicken is cooked through and the vegetables are tender, stirring halfway through cooking.

7. While the chicken fajitas are baking, warm the whole-wheat tortillas according to the package instructions.

8. Once the chicken fajitas are done baking, remove them from the oven and garnish with fresh cilantro if desired.

9. Serve the Baked Chicken Fajitas with Portobello Mushrooms and Whole-Wheat Tortillas hot, along with sliced avocado, Greek yogurt or sour cream, and salsa for topping.

Grilled Herb Chicken with Balsamic Peach Glaze and Quinoa Salad

Ingredients:

For the Grilled Herb Chicken:

- 4 boneless, skinless chicken breasts
- 2 tablespoons olive oil
- 2 cloves garlic, minced
- 1 tablespoon chopped fresh herbs (such as thyme, rosemary, and oregano)
- Salt and pepper to taste

For the Balsamic Peach Glaze:

- 2 ripe peaches, peeled and diced
- 1/4 cup balsamic vinegar
- 2 tablespoons honey
- 1 tablespoon olive oil
- Salt and pepper to taste

For the Quinoa Salad:

- 1 cup quinoa, rinsed
- 2 cups water or low-sodium chicken broth
- 1 cucumber, diced
- 1 bell pepper, diced
- 1/4 cup chopped fresh parsley
- 1/4 cup chopped fresh mint
- Juice of 1 lemon
- 2 tablespoons olive oil
- Salt and pepper to taste

Directions:

1. Preheat the grill to medium-high heat.

2. In a small bowl, whisk together the olive oil, minced garlic, chopped fresh herbs, salt, and pepper. Rub this mixture all over the chicken breasts.

3. In a blender or food processor, combine the diced peaches, balsamic vinegar, honey, olive oil, salt, and pepper. Blend until smooth to make the balsamic peach glaze.

4. Transfer the chicken breasts to the preheated grill and cook for 6-8 minutes per side, or until cooked through and no longer pink in the center. During the last few minutes of grilling, brush the chicken breasts with the balsamic peach glaze, allowing it to caramelize slightly.

5. While the chicken is grilling, prepare the quinoa salad. In a medium saucepan, bring the water or low-sodium chicken broth to a boil. Stir in the quinoa, reduce the heat to low, cover, and simmer for 15-20 minutes, or until the quinoa is cooked and the liquid is absorbed. Remove from heat and let it cool slightly.

6. In a large mixing bowl, combine the cooked quinoa, diced cucumber, diced bell pepper, chopped fresh parsley, chopped fresh mint, lemon juice, olive oil, salt, and pepper. Toss until well combined.

7. Serve the Grilled Herb Chicken with Balsamic Peach Glaze alongside the Quinoa Salad.

Greek Lemon Chicken with Roasted Brussels Sprouts and Whole-Wheat Couscous

Ingredients:

For the Greek Lemon Chicken:

- 4 boneless, skinless chicken breasts
- Juice of 2 lemons
- Zest of 1 lemon
- 2 tablespoons olive oil
- 2 cloves garlic, minced
- 1 teaspoon dried oregano
- 1/2 teaspoon dried thyme
- Salt and pepper to taste

For the Roasted Brussels Sprouts:

- 1 lb Brussels sprouts, trimmed and halved
- 2 tablespoons olive oil
- Salt and pepper to taste

For the Whole-Wheat Couscous:

- 1 cup whole-wheat couscous
- 1 1/4 cups low-sodium chicken broth or water
- 1 tablespoon olive oil
- 1/4 cup chopped fresh parsley
- Salt and pepper to taste

Directions:

1. Preheat the oven to 400°F (200°C).
2. In a small bowl, whisk together the lemon juice, lemon zest, olive oil, minced garlic, dried oregano, dried thyme, salt, and pepper.

3. Place the chicken breasts in a shallow dish and pour the marinade over them. Turn to coat evenly and let them marinate for at least 30 minutes in the refrigerator.

4. While the chicken is marinating, prepare the Brussels sprouts. Place the trimmed and halved Brussels sprouts on a baking sheet. Drizzle with olive oil, season with salt and pepper, and toss to coat evenly. Roast in the preheated oven for 20-25 minutes, or until tender and lightly browned, stirring halfway through cooking.

5. While the Brussels sprouts are roasting, prepare the whole-wheat couscous. In a medium saucepan, bring the low-sodium chicken broth or water to a boil. Stir in the whole-wheat couscous and olive oil. Cover, remove from heat, and let it sit for 5 minutes. Fluff with a fork and stir in the chopped fresh parsley. Season with salt and pepper to taste.

6. While the couscous is cooking, heat a grill pan or skillet over medium-high heat. Remove the chicken breasts from the marinade and discard the excess marinade. Grill the chicken breasts for 6-8 minutes per side, or until cooked through and no longer pink in the center.

7. Serve the Greek Lemon Chicken with Roasted Brussels Sprouts and Whole-Wheat Couscous.

Turkey and Black Bean Burgers with Sweet Potato Buns

Ingredients:

For the Turkey and Black Bean Burgers:
- 1 lb ground turkey
- 1 can (15 oz) black beans, drained and rinsed
- 1/2 cup breadcrumbs (whole-wheat for added fiber)

- 1 small onion, finely chopped
- 2 cloves garlic, minced
- 1 teaspoon ground cumin
- 1 teaspoon chili powder
- 1/2 teaspoon paprika
- Salt and pepper to taste
- 2 tablespoons olive oil (for cooking)

For the Sweet Potato Buns:

- 2 large sweet potatoes
- 2 tablespoons olive oil
- Salt and pepper to taste

For Serving:

- Lettuce leaves
- Sliced tomatoes
- Sliced avocado
- Greek yogurt or light mayo
- Optional toppings: sliced red onion, pickles

Directions:

1. Preheat the oven to 400°F (200°C).
2. Start by making the sweet potato buns. Wash and dry the sweet potatoes, then slice them into rounds, about 1/2 inch thick.
3. Place the sweet potato rounds on a baking sheet lined with parchment paper. Drizzle with olive oil and season with salt and pepper. Toss to coat evenly.
4. Bake the sweet potato rounds in the preheated oven for 20-25 minutes, or until tender and lightly browned, flipping halfway through cooking.

5. While the sweet potato rounds are baking, prepare the turkey and black bean burgers. In a large mixing bowl, combine the ground turkey, drained and rinsed black beans, breadcrumbs, chopped onion, minced garlic, ground cumin, chili powder, paprika, salt, and pepper. Mix until well combined.

6. Divide the mixture into 4 equal portions and shape each portion into a burger patty.

7. Heat the olive oil in a large skillet over medium heat. Add the turkey and black bean burger patties to the skillet and cook for 5-6 minutes per side, or until cooked through and browned on the outside.

8. Once the sweet potato rounds are done baking and the turkey and black bean burgers are cooked through, assemble the burgers. Place a lettuce leaf on top of each sweet potato round, followed by a turkey and black bean burger patty. Top with sliced tomatoes, sliced avocado, and a dollop of Greek yogurt or light mayo. Add any optional toppings if desired.

9. Serve the Turkey and Black Bean Burgers with Sweet Potato Buns immediately.

Chicken Souvlaki Bowls with Greek Yogurt Marinade and Whole-Wheat Pita Bread

Ingredients:

For the Chicken Souvlaki:

- 1 lb boneless, skinless chicken breasts, cut into bite-sized pieces
- 1/4 cup Greek yogurt
- 2 tablespoons olive oil
- 2 cloves garlic, minced

- Juice of 1 lemon

- 1 teaspoon dried oregano

- 1/2 teaspoon dried thyme

- Salt and pepper to taste

For the Greek Salad:

- 2 large tomatoes, diced

- 1 cucumber, diced

- 1/2 red onion, thinly sliced

- 1/4 cup Kalamata olives, pitted and sliced

- 1/4 cup crumbled feta cheese

- 2 tablespoons chopped fresh parsley

- Juice of 1 lemon

- 2 tablespoons olive oil

- Salt and pepper to taste

For Serving:

- Whole-wheat pita bread, warmed

- Tzatziki sauce (optional)

Directions:

1. In a large mixing bowl, combine the Greek yogurt, olive oil, minced garlic, lemon juice, dried oregano, dried thyme, salt, and pepper. Add the bite-sized chicken pieces to the marinade and toss to coat evenly. Cover and refrigerate for at least 30 minutes, or up to 4 hours.

2. While the chicken is marinating, prepare the Greek salad. In a large salad bowl, combine the diced tomatoes, diced cucumber, thinly sliced red onion, sliced Kalamata olives, crumbled feta cheese, and chopped fresh parsley. Drizzle with lemon juice and olive oil, and season with salt and pepper to taste. Toss to combine and set aside.

3. Preheat a grill pan or skillet over medium-high heat. Thread the marinated chicken pieces onto skewers if desired.

4. Grill the chicken skewers or chicken pieces in the preheated grill pan or skillet for 5-6 minutes per side, or until cooked through and lightly charred.

5. While the chicken is grilling, warm the whole-wheat pita bread in the oven or on the stovetop.

6. Once the chicken is cooked through, assemble the Chicken Souvlaki Bowls. Divide the Greek salad among serving bowls, top with the grilled chicken, and serve with warmed whole-wheat pita bread on the side.

7. Optionally, serve with tzatziki sauce on the side for dipping or drizzling over the chicken.

8. Enjoy your delicious and nutritious Chicken Souvlaki Bowls with Greek Yogurt Marinade and Whole-Wheat Pita Bread!

Sheet-Pan Teriyaki Salmon with Roasted Vegetables and Quinoa

Ingredients:

For the Teriyaki Salmon:

- 4 salmon filets
- 1/4 cup low-sodium soy sauce or tamari
- 2 tablespoons honey or maple syrup
- 2 tablespoons rice vinegar
- 1 tablespoon sesame oil
- 2 cloves garlic, minced
- 1 teaspoon grated ginger

- 1 tablespoon cornstarch
- 2 tablespoons water
- Sesame seeds for garnish (optional)
- Sliced green onions for garnish (optional)

For the Roasted Vegetables:

- 2 cups chopped vegetables (such as bell peppers, broccoli, carrots, and snap peas)
- 1 tablespoon olive oil
- Salt and pepper to taste

For the Quinoa:

- 1 cup quinoa, rinsed
- 2 cups water or low-sodium chicken broth
- Salt to taste

Directions:

1. Preheat the oven to 400°F (200°C). Line a baking sheet with parchment paper or lightly grease it with olive oil.

2. In a small saucepan, combine the low-sodium soy sauce or tamari, honey or maple syrup, rice vinegar, sesame oil, minced garlic, and grated ginger. Heat over medium heat until the mixture starts to simmer.

3. In a small bowl, whisk together the cornstarch and water until smooth. Stir the cornstarch slurry into the saucepan with the simmering sauce. Cook, stirring constantly, until the sauce thickens, about 2-3 minutes. Remove from heat and set aside.

4. Place the salmon filets on the prepared baking sheet. Brush the salmon filets generously with the teriyaki sauce, reserving some sauce for serving. Sprinkle sesame seeds over the salmon filets if desired.

5. In a large mixing bowl, toss the chopped vegetables with olive oil, salt, and pepper until evenly coated. Spread the vegetables out on the baking sheet around the salmon filets.

6. Roast in the preheated oven for 12-15 minutes, or until the salmon is cooked through and the vegetables are tender and lightly browned, stirring the vegetables halfway through cooking.

7. While the salmon and vegetables are roasting, prepare the quinoa. In a medium saucepan, bring the water or low-sodium chicken broth to a boil. Stir in the rinsed quinoa and salt to taste. Cover, reduce the heat to low, and simmer for 15-20 minutes, or until the quinoa is cooked and the liquid is absorbed. Remove from heat and let it sit, covered, for 5 minutes. Fluff with a fork.

8. Serve the Sheet-Pan Teriyaki Salmon with Roasted Vegetables and Quinoa, drizzling any remaining teriyaki sauce over the salmon filets.

9. Garnish with sliced green onions if desired.

10. Enjoy your delicious and nutritious meal!

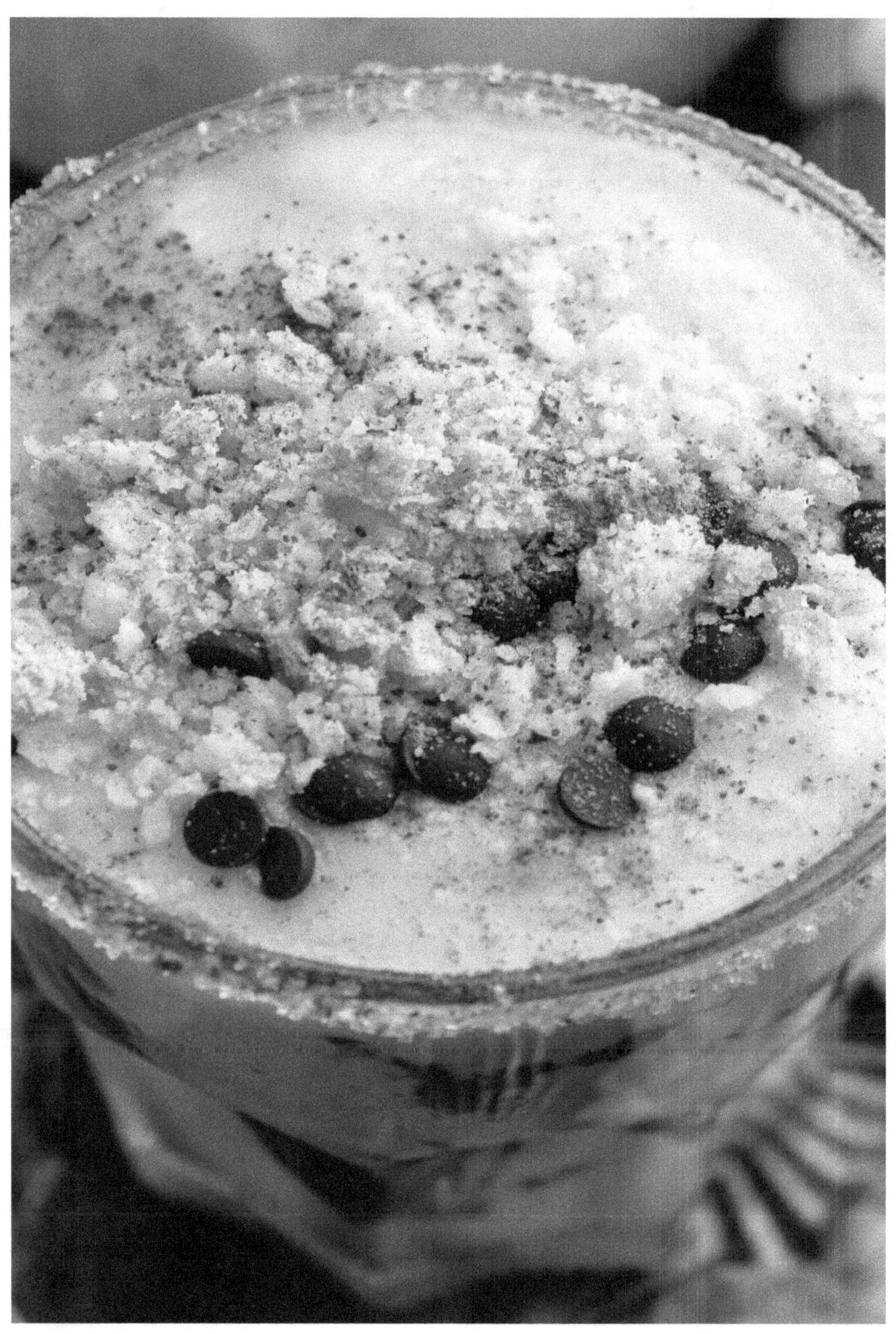

Chapter 13: Smoothie Recipes

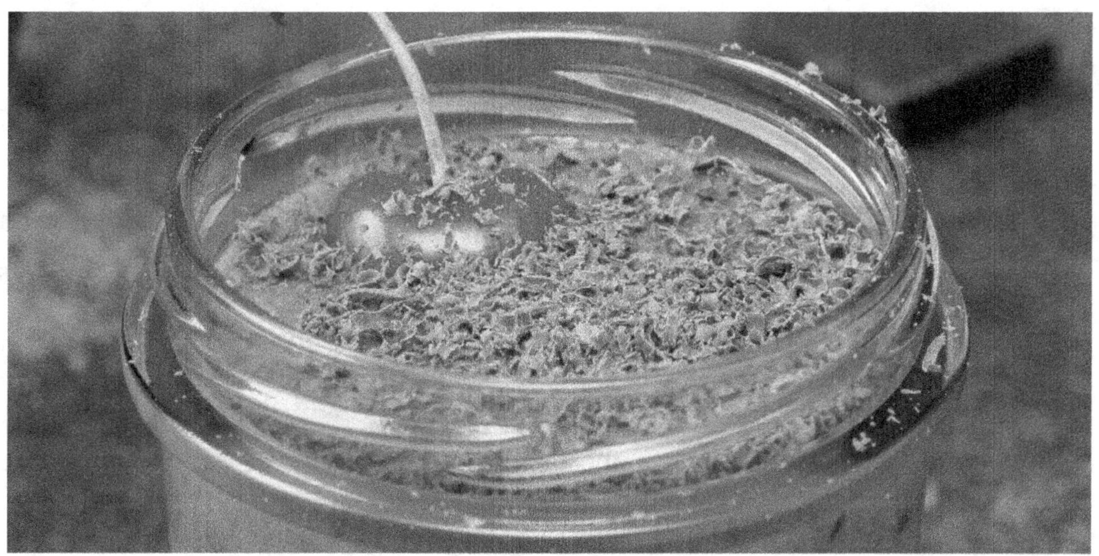

Chocolate Cherry Smoothie

Ingredients:

- 1 cup unsweetened almond milk
- 1/2 cup frozen cherries
- 1 tablespoon unsweetened cocoa powder
- 1/2 ripe banana
- 1 tablespoon chia seeds (optional)
- 1 tablespoon almond butter (unsweetened)
- Ice cubes (optional)

Directions:

1. In a blender, combine the unsweetened almond milk, frozen cherries, unsweetened cocoa powder, ripe banana, chia seeds (if using), and almond butter.

2. Blend the ingredients until smooth and creamy. If the smoothie is too thick, you can add a little more almond milk to reach your desired consistency.

3. If desired, add a few ice cubes to the blender and blend again to make the smoothie colder.

4. Taste the smoothie and adjust the sweetness if necessary. If you prefer a sweeter smoothie, you can add a small amount of sweetener such as stevia or a teaspoon of honey or maple syrup. Keep in mind that it's best to limit added sugars for managing diabetes, so adjust accordingly.

5. Once you're satisfied with the taste and consistency, pour the smoothie into a glass and enjoy immediately.

Green Machine Smoothie

Ingredients:
- 1 cup spinach leaves, tightly packed
- 1/2 ripe avocado
- 1/2 cucumber, peeled and chopped
- 1/2 green apple, cored and chopped
- 1/2 cup unsweetened almond milk
- 1 tablespoon chia seeds (optional)
- Juice of 1/2 lemon
- Ice cubes (optional)

Directions:
1. In a blender, combine the spinach leaves, ripe avocado, chopped cucumber, chopped green apple, unsweetened almond milk, and chia seeds (if using).

2. Squeeze the juice of half a lemon into the blender.

3. Blend the ingredients until smooth and creamy. If the smoothie is too thick, you can add a little more almond milk to reach your desired consistency.

4. If desired, add a few ice cubes to the blender and blend again to make the smoothie colder.

5. Taste the smoothie and adjust the flavor if necessary. If you prefer a sweeter smoothie, you can add a small amount of sweetener such as stevia or a teaspoon of honey or maple syrup. Keep in mind that it's best to limit added sugars for managing diabetes, so adjust accordingly.

6. Once you're satisfied with the taste and consistency, pour the smoothie into a glass and enjoy immediately.

Pumpkin Spice Smoothie

Ingredients:
- 1/2 cup unsweetened canned pumpkin puree
- 1/2 ripe banana
- 1/2 cup unsweetened almond milk
- 1/2 teaspoon ground cinnamon
- 1/4 teaspoon ground nutmeg
- 1/4 teaspoon ground ginger
- 1/4 teaspoon ground cloves
- 1 tablespoon chia seeds (optional)
- 1 tablespoon unsweetened almond butter
- Ice cubes (optional)

Directions:

1. In a blender, combine the canned pumpkin puree, ripe banana, unsweetened almond milk, ground cinnamon, ground nutmeg, ground ginger, ground cloves, chia seeds (if using), and unsweetened almond butter.

2. Blend the ingredients until smooth and creamy. If the smoothie is too thick, you can add a little more almond milk to reach your desired consistency.

3. If desired, add a few ice cubes to the blender and blend again to make the smoothie colder.

4. Taste the smoothie and adjust the flavor if necessary. If you prefer a sweeter smoothie, you can add a small amount of sweetener such as stevia or a teaspoon of honey or maple syrup. Keep in mind that it's best to limit added sugars for managing diabetes, so adjust accordingly.

5. Once you're satisfied with the taste and consistency, pour the smoothie into a glass and enjoy immediately.

Tropical Green Smoothie

Ingredients:

- 1 cup spinach leaves, tightly packed
- 1/2 cup frozen pineapple chunks
- 1/2 cup frozen mango chunks
- 1/2 ripe banana
- 1/2 cup unsweetened coconut milk
- 1 tablespoon chia seeds (optional)
- Juice of 1/2 lime
- Ice cubes (optional)

Directions:

1. In a blender, combine the spinach leaves, frozen pineapple chunks, frozen mango chunks, ripe banana, unsweetened coconut milk, and chia seeds (if using).

2. Squeeze the juice of half a lime into the blender.

3. Blend the ingredients until smooth and creamy. If the smoothie is too thick, you can add a little more coconut milk to reach your desired consistency.

4. If desired, add a few ice cubes to the blender and blend again to make the smoothie colder.

5. Taste the smoothie and adjust the flavor if necessary. If you prefer a sweeter smoothie, you can add a small amount of sweetener such as stevia or a teaspoon of honey or maple syrup. Keep in mind that it's best to limit added sugars for managing diabetes, so adjust accordingly.

6. Once you're satisfied with the taste and consistency, pour the smoothie into a glass and enjoy immediately.

Coffee Cooler Smoothie

Ingredients:

- 1/2 cup brewed coffee, chilled
- 1/2 cup unsweetened almond milk
- 1/2 ripe banana
- 1 tablespoon unsweetened cocoa powder
- 1 tablespoon almond butter (unsweetened)
- 1/2 teaspoon vanilla extract
- Ice cubes (optional)

Directions:

1. Brew your favorite coffee and allow it to cool to room temperature or chill it in the refrigerator for a cold smoothie.
2. In a blender, combine the brewed coffee, unsweetened almond milk, ripe banana, unsweetened cocoa powder, almond butter, and vanilla extract.
3. Add ice cubes if you want a colder smoothie.
4. Blend the ingredients until smooth and creamy. If the smoothie is too thick, you can add a little more almond milk to reach your desired consistency.
5. Taste the smoothie and adjust the flavor if necessary. If you prefer a sweeter smoothie, you can add a small amount of sweetener such as stevia or a teaspoon of honey or maple syrup. Keep in mind that it's best to limit added sugars for managing diabetes, so adjust accordingly.
6. Once you're satisfied with the taste and consistency, pour the smoothie into a glass and enjoy immediately.

Carrot Cake Smoothie

Ingredients:

- 1 medium carrot, peeled and chopped
- 1/2 cup cooked, cooled cauliflower florets
- 1/2 ripe banana
- 1/4 cup unsweetened almond milk
- 1/4 cup plain Greek yogurt
- 1 tablespoon unsweetened shredded coconut
- 1 tablespoon chopped walnuts
- 1/2 teaspoon ground cinnamon

- 1/4 teaspoon ground nutmeg
- 1/4 teaspoon ground ginger
- 1 tablespoon chia seeds (optional)
- Ice cubes (optional)

Directions:

1. In a blender, combine the chopped carrot, cooked cauliflower florets, ripe banana, unsweetened almond milk, plain Greek yogurt, unsweetened shredded coconut, chopped walnuts, ground cinnamon, ground nutmeg, and ground ginger.
2. If using chia seeds, add them to the blender as well.
3. Add ice cubes if you want a colder smoothie.
4. Blend the ingredients until smooth and creamy. If the smoothie is too thick, you can add a little more almond milk to reach your desired consistency.
5. Taste the smoothie and adjust the flavor if necessary. If you prefer a sweeter smoothie, you can add a small amount of sweetener such as stevia or a teaspoon of honey or maple syrup. Keep in mind that it's best to limit added sugars for managing diabetes, so adjust accordingly.
6. Once you're satisfied with the taste and consistency, pour the smoothie into a glass and enjoy immediately.

Watermelon Mint Cooler

Ingredients:

- 2 cups cubed seedless watermelon
- 1/4 cup fresh mint leaves
- Juice of 1 lime
- 1 cup unsweetened coconut water

- Ice cubes (optional)
- Mint leaves and watermelon wedges for garnish (optional)

Directions:

1. In a blender, combine the cubed watermelon, fresh mint leaves, lime juice, and unsweetened coconut water.
2. If you prefer a colder drink, add a few ice cubes to the blender.
3. Blend the ingredients until smooth and well combined.
4. Taste the cooler and adjust the flavor if necessary. If you prefer it sweeter, you can add a small amount of sweetener like stevia or honey, but keep in mind to limit added sugars for managing diabetes.
5. Once you're satisfied with the taste, pour the cooler into glasses.
6. Garnish each glass with a sprig of mint leaves and a watermelon wedge if desired.
7. Serve immediately and enjoy this refreshing Watermelon Mint Cooler!

Pear and Ginger Smoothie

Ingredients:

- 1 ripe pear, cored and chopped
- 1/2 inch piece of fresh ginger, peeled and grated
- 1/2 cup plain Greek yogurt
- 1/2 cup unsweetened almond milk
- 1 tablespoon chia seeds (optional)
- 1 teaspoon honey or maple syrup (optional, adjust to taste)
- Ice cubes (optional)

Directions:

1. In a blender, combine the chopped pear, grated ginger, plain Greek yogurt, unsweetened almond milk, and chia seeds (if using).

2. Add honey or maple syrup if you prefer a sweeter smoothie, but keep in mind to limit added sugars for managing diabetes.

3. Add ice cubes if you prefer a colder smoothie.

4. Blend the ingredients until smooth and creamy. If the smoothie is too thick, you can add a little more almond milk to reach your desired consistency.

5. Taste the smoothie and adjust the sweetness or ginger flavor if necessary.

6. Once you're satisfied with the taste and consistency, pour the smoothie into glasses.

7. Serve immediately and enjoy this delicious Pear and Ginger Smoothie!

Matcha Green Tea Smoothie

Ingredients:

- 1 teaspoon matcha green tea powder
- 1 ripe banana, frozen
- 1/2 cup plain Greek yogurt
- 1/2 cup unsweetened almond milk
- 1 tablespoon chia seeds (optional)
- 1 teaspoon honey or maple syrup (optional, adjust to taste)
- Ice cubes (optional)

Directions:

1. In a blender, combine the matcha green tea powder, frozen banana, plain Greek yogurt, unsweetened almond milk, and chia seeds (if using).

2. Add honey or maple syrup if you prefer a sweeter smoothie, but keep in mind to limit added sugars for managing diabetes.

3. Add ice cubes if you prefer a colder smoothie.

4. Blend the ingredients until smooth and creamy. If the smoothie is too thick, you can add a little more almond milk to reach your desired consistency.

5. Taste the smoothie and adjust the sweetness if necessary.

6. Once you're satisfied with the taste and consistency, pour the smoothie into glasses.

7. Serve immediately and enjoy this refreshing Matcha Green Tea Smoothie!

Very Berry Chia Smoothie

Ingredients:

- 1/2 cup mixed berries (such as strawberries, blueberries, raspberries)
- 1/2 ripe banana, frozen
- 1 tablespoon chia seeds
- 1/2 cup plain Greek yogurt
- 1/2 cup unsweetened almond milk
- 1 teaspoon honey or maple syrup (optional, adjust to taste)
- Ice cubes (optional)

Directions:

1. In a blender, combine the mixed berries, frozen banana, chia seeds, plain Greek yogurt, unsweetened almond milk, and honey or maple syrup (if using).

2. Add ice cubes if you prefer a colder smoothie.

3. Blend the ingredients until smooth and creamy. If the smoothie is too thick, you can add a little more almond milk to reach your desired consistency.

4. Taste the smoothie and adjust the sweetness if necessary.

5. Once you're satisfied with the taste and consistency, pour the smoothie into glasses.

6. Serve immediately and enjoy this delicious Very Berry Chia Smoothie!

Sweet Greens and Peach Perfection

Ingredients:

- 1 ripe peach, pitted and chopped
- 1 cup spinach leaves, tightly packed
- 1/2 ripe banana, frozen
- 1/2 cup unsweetened almond milk
- 1 tablespoon chia seeds
- 1 teaspoon honey or maple syrup (optional, adjust to taste)
- Ice cubes (optional)

Directions:

1. In a blender, combine the chopped peach, spinach leaves, frozen banana, unsweetened almond milk, chia seeds, and honey or maple syrup (if using).

2. Add ice cubes if you prefer a colder smoothie.

3. Blend the ingredients until smooth and creamy. If the smoothie is too thick, you can add a little more almond milk to reach your desired consistency.

4. Taste the smoothie and adjust the sweetness if necessary.

5. Once you're satisfied with the taste and consistency, pour the smoothie into glasses.

6. Serve immediately and enjoy this refreshing Sweet Greens and Peach Perfection Smoothie!

Creamy Avocado and Mango Magic

Ingredients:

- 1/2 ripe avocado, peeled and pitted
- 1/2 cup chopped ripe mango
- 1/2 cup plain Greek yogurt
- 1/2 cup unsweetened almond milk
- 1 tablespoon chia seeds
- 1 teaspoon honey or maple syrup (optional, adjust to taste)
- Ice cubes (optional)

Directions:

1. In a blender, combine the ripe avocado, chopped mango, plain Greek yogurt, unsweetened almond milk, chia seeds, and honey or maple syrup (if using).
2. Add ice cubes if you prefer a colder smoothie.
3. Blend the ingredients until smooth and creamy. If the smoothie is too thick, you can add a little more almond milk to reach your desired consistency.
4. Taste the smoothie and adjust the sweetness if necessary.
5. Once you're satisfied with the taste and consistency, pour the smoothie into glasses.
6. Serve immediately and enjoy this delicious Creamy Avocado and Mango Magic Smoothie!

High-Fiber Fig and Flax Delight

Ingredients:

- 2 dried figs, stems removed and chopped

- 1 tablespoon ground flaxseeds
- 1/2 cup plain Greek yogurt
- 1/2 cup unsweetened almond milk
- 1 tablespoon almond butter (unsweetened)
- 1 teaspoon honey or maple syrup (optional, adjust to taste)
- Ice cubes (optional)

Directions:

1. In a blender, combine the chopped dried figs, ground flaxseeds, plain Greek yogurt, unsweetened almond milk, almond butter, and honey or maple syrup (if using).
2. Add ice cubes if you prefer a colder smoothie.
3. Blend the ingredients until smooth and creamy. If the smoothie is too thick, you can add a little more almond milk to reach your desired consistency.
4. Taste the smoothie and adjust the sweetness if necessary.
5. Once you're satisfied with the taste and consistency, pour the smoothie into glasses.
6. Serve immediately and enjoy this nutritious High-Fiber Fig and Flax Delight Smoothie!

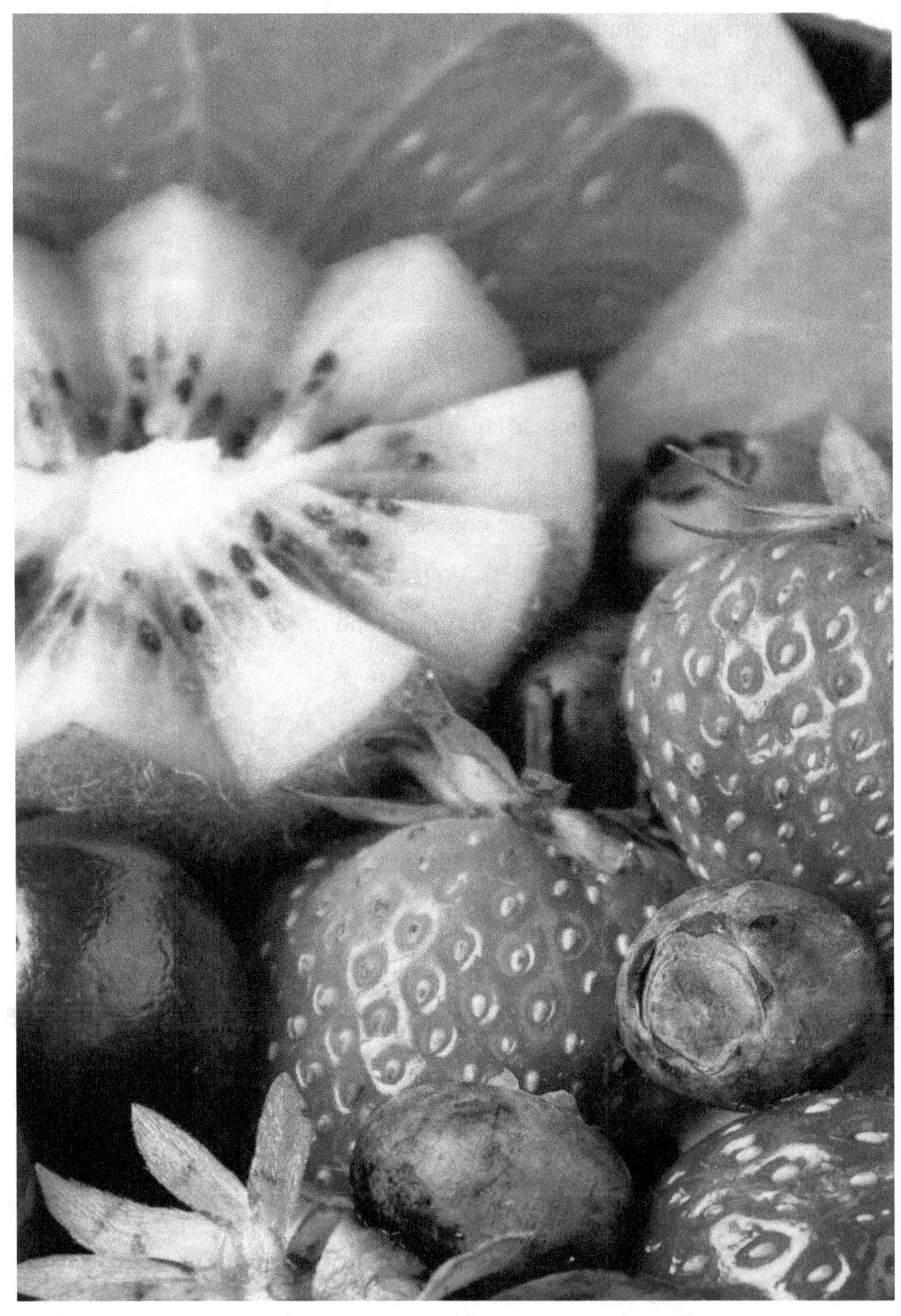

Chapter 14: 21-Day Exercise Plan for Women

Regular physical activity is crucial for managing Type 2 diabetes in women. Exercise helps improve insulin sensitivity, lowers blood sugar levels, reduces body fat, and enhances overall well-being. This 21-day exercise plan is designed specifically for women with Type 2 diabetes to incorporate physical activity into their daily routine and achieve better diabetes management.

Week 1: Building Foundation

Day 1-3: Walking Routine

- Aim for 20-30 minutes of brisk walking each day.
- Start with a comfortable pace and gradually increase speed.
- Monitor blood sugar levels before and after walking to understand its impact.

Day 4: Strength Training

- Begin with bodyweight exercises like squats, lunges, push-ups, and planks.
- Perform 2 sets of 10-12 repetitions for each exercise.
- Focus on proper form and controlled movements.

Day 5-7: Yoga and Stretching

- Practice gentle yoga poses and stretches to improve flexibility and reduce stress.

- Include poses like downward dog, child's pose, and seated spinal twist.
- Pay attention to breathing and relaxation techniques.

Week 2: Increasing Intensity

Day 8-10: Cardio Workouts

- Incorporate 30-40 minutes of cardiovascular exercises such as cycling, swimming, or dancing.
- Maintain a moderate intensity level, where you can still hold a conversation but feel slightly breathless.
- Adjust the intensity based on your fitness level and comfort.

Day 11: Interval Training

- Try interval training by alternating between periods of high intensity and low intensity.
- For example, alternate between 1 minute of fast walking or jogging and 2 minutes of walking at a moderate pace.
- Aim for 20-25 minutes of intervals.

Day 12-14: Pilates

- Engage in Pilates exercises to strengthen core muscles and improve posture.
- Focus on movements that target abdominal muscles, back, and pelvic floor.
- Perform controlled movements with proper alignment.

Week 3: Enhancing Endurance

Day 15-17: Aerobic Exercise

- Engage in longer sessions of aerobic exercises like running, cycling, or swimming.
- Gradually increase the duration to 45-60 minutes per session.
- Monitor blood sugar levels before, during, and after exercise to prevent hypoglycemia.

Day 18: Circuit Training

- Combine strength training and cardiovascular exercises into a circuit workout.
- Perform 1 minute of each exercise with minimal rest in between.
- Include exercises like squats, lunges, jumping jacks, and push-ups.

Day 19-21: Active Recreation

- Incorporate enjoyable physical activities such as hiking, dancing, or playing sports.
- Invite friends or family members to join to make it more fun and social.
- Focus on activities that you genuinely enjoy to stay motivated.

Tips for Success:

1. Stay hydrated before, during, and after exercise.
2. Wear comfortable and supportive footwear.
3. Monitor blood sugar levels regularly, especially when trying new exercises or intensities.
4. Listen to your body and modify exercises as needed to avoid injury.

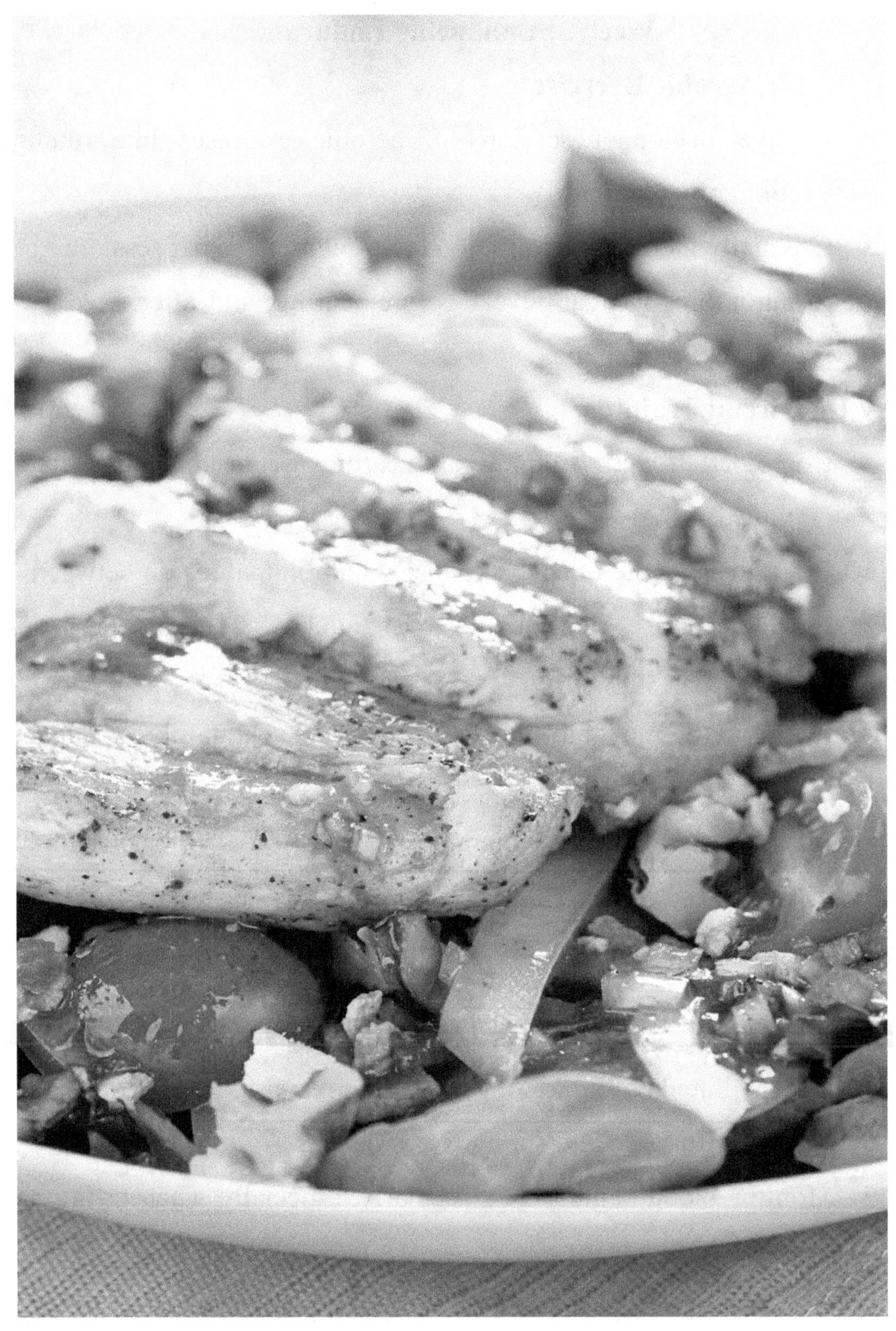

Conclusion

Congratulations on taking charge of your health! Throughout this book, you've learned important facts about type 2 diabetes, how to control it with food, and how to prepare tasty dishes to improve your health.

Remember you are not alone in this. Millions of individuals with type 2 diabetes have meaningful lives. Food is a strong instrument, therefore maintaining good eating habits will help manage your blood sugar and general well-being.

Embrace a Healthy Lifestyle:
- To achieve the best blood sugar management, combine good nutrition with frequent exercise.
- Prioritize enough sleep for general health and well-being.
- Reduce stress using relaxation practices such as yoga or meditation.
- Schedule frequent check-ups with your doctor to assess your progress and change your treatment plan as required.

Living with type 2 diabetes is a journey, not a destination. Making informed decisions about your nutrition, exercise, and lifestyle can allow you to properly manage your illness and enjoy a long, healthy, and meaningful life.

Best wishes on your road to a healthy you!

"I embrace the opportunity to explore new flavors and nourish my body with the vibrant recipes in this cookbook, knowing they support my blood sugar management."

"Each meal I create from this cookbook is a celebration of my commitment to self-care and well-being."

"I am grateful for the abundance of delicious, diabetes-friendly options available to me, allowing me to enjoy a diverse and satisfying diet."

"With every bite, I am fueling my body with the nutrients it needs to thrive, and I feel empowered by the positive choices I make for my health."

"I trust in my ability to adapt and find joy in the journey of discovering new ways to support my blood sugar levels through wholesome, flavorful meals."

"Every recipe I try brings me closer to achieving my health goals, and I approach each cooking experience with enthusiasm and curiosity."

"I am worthy of investing time and effort into caring for my health, and preparing meals from this cookbook is a loving act of self-respect."

"As I savor each bite, I affirm my commitment to prioritizing my well-being and nurturing my body with nourishing foods."